2003

Setting Limits Fairly

Setting Limits Fairly

Can We Learn to Share Medical Resources?

Norman Daniels
James E. Sabin

OXFORD
UNIVERSITY PRESS

2002

OXFORD
UNIVERSITY PRESS

Oxford   New York
Auckland   Bangkok   Buenos Aires   Cape Town   Chennai
Dar es Salaam   Delhi   Hong Kong   Istanbul   Karachi   Kolkata
Kuala Lumpur   Madrid   Melbourne   Mexico City   Mumbai   Nairobi
São Paulo   Shanghai   Singapore   Taipei   Tokyo   Toronto

and an associated company in Berlin

Library of Congress Cataloging-in-Publication Data
Daniels, Norman, 1942-
Settings limits fairly : can we learn to share medical resources? /
Norman Daniels, James E. Sabin.
p. cm.
Includes bibliographical references and index.
ISBN 0-19-514936-X
1. Medical care—Social aspects. 2. Medical economics—Moral and ethical aspects.
3. Right to health care.
I. Sabin, James E. II. Title.
RA445.D33 2002   362.1′042—dc21   2001047458

1 2 3 4 5 6 7 8 9

Printed in the United States of America
on acid-free paper.

For Anne and Margery

Preface

Our goal in this book is to answer a central question about justice and health care: how can a society or health plan meet population health care needs fairly under resource limitations? Because resources are limited, all societies must set limits to care and establish priorities about how resources will be used—whether they acknowledge doing so or not. Limit setting is often greeted with distrust and with challenges to the moral authority, or legitimacy, of those who set the limits. This is true in the mixed, public and private, nonuniversal coverage system we have in the United States—where it is perceived as a backlash against managed care. But it is also true in highly egalitarian, universal coverage systems in advanced economies, just as it is in developing countries struggling with more severe limits on resources.

Though we agree on the central importance of this question, we come to it from different directions, having taken very different routes in our careers. One of us, James Sabin, is a psychiatrist who has treated patients for 35 years. He has also served for a time as associate medical director of a health maintenance organization (HMO), and he is currently director of the ethics program at Harvard Pilgrim Health Care. He has struggled with the challenge of advocating for patients in a system that cares for a population of patients within an overall budget. Both as manager and clinician, he has faced the challenge of reconciling individual patient needs and responsibilities to individual patients with concerns about population health. For him, our central question must have a practical answer. It must help guide clinical practice as well as the organization within which clinicians' skills are organized to benefit patients.

The other of us, Norman Daniels, is a philosopher. He has treated no patients and managed no delivery systems. He has, however, thought about problems of justice for over 30 years and has worked specifically on justice and health policy for most of that time. He was led to our question because he was dissatisfied with how theories of justice—including his own work on just health care—failed to guide adequately the decisions with which Jim Sabin and others like him grappled. For him, the answer to our central question must not only be practical but must also rest squarely on defensible moral foundations. The guidance it offers clinicians and organizations must withstand rigorous philosophical challenge.

However different the routes that led us to this question, in this book we walk a common path. We offer a practical, yet theoretically defensible, account of how societies should set limits to and priorities for health care. Put less euphemistically, we explain how to ration fairly. If we are right, our answer will tell us how we can learn to share medical resources.

Both of us have worked actively to seek universal health care coverage in the United States. We have long seen this as the most urgent issue of justice facing the health care system in the United States. More specifically, we have both argued for, worked for, and continued to favor a single-payer form of financing the American system. In other writings we have decried the way in which the bad may drive out the good in our system of delivery, where employers buy the services of health plans largely on the basis of price, not quality.

Why then do we build our account of how to ration fairly out of examples drawn in part from practices in such an unjust and inefficient national system, especially one in which managed care is continuously evolving, not always for the better? Our answer is that rationing fairly is something that ought to be done in systems whether or not they are in other ways unjust or badly organized. We have aimed for an account that will give guidance in both non-ideal and more ideal systems.

In what follows we speak to many different audiences struggling in their own ways with our central question: patients who may be denied specific treatments, clinicians whose patients may not be covered for treatments they want to provide, managers in public agencies and private health plans who want to deliver quality care under resource limits, a public that is alarmed at the gap between what the media and the internet tell it is possible and what a system they may distrust delivers, and policy makers and politicians who may publicly duck the question of rationing fairly but who must address it nevertheless.

The answer we offer to all these audiences is not just wishful theorizing. Many institutions, in the United States and abroad, have been groping toward the answer we describe, experimenting with aspects of it, providing material for social learning about it. By framing their experience within our answer to the question, we hope to provide coherence and direction to what has been explored only piecemeal and empirically.

We base our answer on collaborative research spanning more than a decade and involving many individuals and institutions to which we owe thanks. A number of foundations have supported our work in this period. We gratefully acknowledge the generosity of the Greenwall Foundation, whose early support helped us to launch the decade-long project, and whose continued confidence and support has helped us carry it through to this point; the Robert Wood Johnson Foundation, which contributed to several stages of our joint work, and which also provided Norman Daniels with a Robert Wood Johnson Investigator Award during 1998–2001; the National Science Foundation; the Retirement Research Foundation; the Substance Abuse and Mental Health Services Agency; the Harvard Pilgrim Health Care Foundation; the Medicine as a Profession Program of the Open Society Institute; and, more recently, the Merck Company Foundation. Norman Daniels also was supported in 1999–2000 by a Tufts sabbatical grant and, in 2000–2001 by a senior fellowship at the NIH Clinical Bioethics Center.

We also gratefully acknowledge the help of particular collaborating institutions. In our empirical work, we have viewed the institutions we study as collaborators, not simply research subjects, seeking mutual learning from the interaction. We thank Harvard Pilgrim Health Care for the detailed access it gave us to meetings and videotapes of its Committee on Appropriate Technology. We thank as well Aetna, the Blue Cross Blue Shield Technology Evaluation Center, California Blue Shield, Group Health Cooperative of Puget Sound, Health Partners of Minnesota, Kaiser Permanente of Northern California, Massachusetts Behavioral Health Partnership, Merit Behavioral Care of Iowa, Oregon Blue Cross Blue Shield, the Oregon Health Resources Commission and PacifiCare.

We also thank many individuals who have offered us criticism and support for our pursuing these ideas over a long period of time: Laurie Ansorge-Ball, Naomi Aronson, Blair Beebe, Marc Berger, Jack Bryant, Dan Brock, Allen Buchanan, Bruce Bullen, Daniel Callahan, Carolyn Clancy, Josh Cohen, Nancy Collins, Joel Cooper, Joan Discher, Joseph Dorsey, Ezekiel Emanuel, Rob Epstein, David Estlund, Len Fleck, Larry Gottlieb, Gwen Halaas, Chris Ham, Dan Harris, Chris Hennessy, Frances Kamm, Nancy Lane, John Ludden, Al Martin, Bill McGivney, David Mechanic, Gordon Moore, Peggy O'Kane, Steven Pearson, Lisa Raiola, Sim Rubenstein, Lawrence Sager, John Santa, Linda Shelton, Richard Sheola, Mona Simons, Peter Singer and his colleagues at University of Toronto Bioethics Center, William Stubing, Mitchell Sugarman, Russell Teagarden, Dennis Thompson, and Dan Wikler. We thank Roxanne Fay, Melinda Karp and Susann Wilkenson, who at different times were part of our research team.

Finally, we owe thanks for permission to draw on previously published material in writing this book. Specifically, in Chapters 3 and 4 we have drawn on our article, "Limits to Health Care: Fair Procedures, Democratic Deliberation, and the

Legitimacy Problem for Insurers," in *Philosophy and Public Affairs* (1997) and in Chapter 5, from our "Last-chance therapies and managed care: Pluralism, fair procedures, and legitimacy," in *Hastings Center Report* (1998). In Chapter 10 we have used material from James Sabin's "Fairness as a problem of love and the heart: a clinician's perspective on priority setting," in the *British Medical Journal* (1998).

We also wish to acknowledge the intellectual precursor to our title, Daniel Callahan's "Setting Limits: Medical Goals in an Aging Society" (Callahan, 1987). Although Callahan focused primarily on the competition for medical resources between the old and the young, his title has become a common way to refer to the broader issue of setting priorities and rationing health care.

Medford, Massachusetts   N.D.
Boston, Massachusetts   J.S.

Contents

Setting Limits Fairly

1

OUR LIVES IN WHOSE HANDS?

LIMITS AND LEGITIMACY

All societies set limits to health care one way or another, fairly or unfairly.

The need for societal limits, and the problem of how to set them, first emerged in the last half of the 20th century. In the early 1900s, medical care was delivered mainly by the solo doctor out of his head, hands, and little black bag. Medical services had little effect on the course of most illness, and no one else except family members had much of a stake or interest in the transaction between the doctor and his patient. The issue of limits did not arise.

As medical knowledge and technology advanced, especially after World War II, and even more so in the last 30 years, health care came to be produced by a complex system of scientists, practitioners, corporations, hospitals, and other delivery institutions. With this change, health care became a far more effective, but far more costly, means of improving individual and population health. As a result, the many stakeholders involved in the production of health care, as well as the whole population to which it is delivered, now have an interest in how this valuable resource is used and distributed.

The major force driving up health care costs worldwide is the emergence of new technologies, including new procedures, drugs, devices, and diagnostic techniques. Aging populations and increased expectations about what medicine can and should do for us mean there is ever increasing demand for what technology makes pos-

1

sible, and rapid technological progress unrelentingly expands what is possible. As a result, the problem of limiting care in a fair and socially acceptable way is arguably the most important—and divisive—issue facing the design of medical delivery systems in the next century. This is true not only in wealthy systems, where the public has some control over what counts as "reasonable" scarcity, but in poorer developing countries as well where resource scarcity is extreme but better-off classes demand all the benefits medicine can offer. Limits are the price of medical success, not medical failure.

Justice requires that all societies meet health care needs fairly under reasonable resource constraints. Of course, a just health care system should use its resources wisely, avoiding waste and aiming to get value for the money spent on health care. But even a wealthy country with a highly efficient health care system will have to set limits to—in other words, ration—the health care it guarantees everyone. However important, health care—by which we refer broadly to preventive, curative, rehabilitative and social support services for physical and mental illness, and disability—is not the only important social good. Societies must also provide education, jobs, transportation, energy, defense, research, art and culture, and well-functioning government and political institutions. Society simply cannot meet all medical needs, and certainly not all medical preferences, so it must decide which needs should be given priority and when resources are better spent elsewhere.

How should decisions about such limits be made? In this book, we propose a practical approach to this problem, one that addresses the common issue of limit setting in the United States and elsewhere.

Our task would be much simpler if people could agree on principles of distributive justice that would determine how to set fair limits to health care. If societies agreed on such principles, it would be possible to check decisions about health care limits against them. If the proposed limits conformed with these principles, they would stand. If the limits failed to conform, they would be judged unjust and changed. Disagreements about the fairness of actual limit-setting decisions would either be about how to interpret the distributive principles or about the facts of the situation. Many societies have well-established and reliable, if imperfect, legal procedures for resolving such disputes about facts and interpretations.

Unfortunately, no democratic society we are aware of has achieved consensus on such distributive principles for health care. Even people who want to cooperate in steering a society's health system will hold diverse moral and religious views. Their individual value systems will lead them to disagree morally about what constitutes a fair allocation of resources to meet competing health care needs. Nevertheless, despite these disagreements, societies must arrive at social policies.

As an example of a crucial challenge for every health system that principles do not solve, consider the issue we call the "Priorities Problem" (Daniels, 1993, 1998a). How much priority should a society give to its most seriously ill patients? What does society owe such worst-off patients?

One view would be to give the sickest patients complete priority. This is not a hypothetical position. In the mid 1990s, the Swedish Parliamentary Priorities Commission (1995) asserted that a first principle of distribution should be to help the most vulnerable and seriously ill. Giving such priority to the sickest patients, however, often means sacrificing the greater health benefits medicine might deliver to less seriously ill patients. Some seriously ill patients may be so ill that they do not respond well to treatments like organ transplants or chemotherapy. The initial Swedish approach gave priority to the sickest no matter how much their treatment cost or how small the benefit they received. Many people, however, think that giving strict priority to the sickest is unjustifiable when it means sacrificing substantially greater benefits for others.

Another view is that society should maximize the total benefit its health care expenditures provide, regardless of who gets those benefits. This view gives no special priority to the most seriously ill. This too is not a hypothetical position. When Oregon first began to set priorities among services received by Medicaid patients in the beginning of the 1990s, it ranked all services by their relative cost-effectiveness. The initial Oregon approach gave no priority to the sickest patients. Its aim was to get the most benefit from every dollar spent in the Medicaid program.

Giving no priority to the sickest, however, violates the strong moral concern many people feel for the most vulnerable among us. When the consequences of the Oregon plan became apparent—in its initial priority ranking, capping teeth had a higher priority than surgery for appendicitis—the public and the state commissioners establishing priorities rejected this approach (Hadorn, 1991). They adopted instead a method that gave some priority to more seriously ill patients.

The lessons from Oregon and Sweden are quite general: Most people will neither sacrifice everything to the sickest, nor abandon them.

How about something in between? Most would agree to giving the sickest patients some, but not complete, priority. This middle range is what most health care systems end up incorporating into their resource allocation decisions. But this middle-range priority is messy. Just how much priority should the sickest get? Where in the middle should the lines be drawn? Unlike giving complete priority (the initial Swedish position) or no priority (the initial Oregon position), giving "some" priority is quite indeterminate. Adopting a middle position means that there may be several fair and politically acceptable policy alternatives.

The problem with setting limits is not simply that we currently lack a consensus on principles that would tell us how to distribute health care fairly. Even if such a consensus is achievable, it is not likely to be soon. Societies such as Sweden, Denmark, Norway, and the Netherlands that have established national commissions to articulate a public agreement on such principles have found that moral disagreement continues to disrupt the smooth functioning of limit-setting decisions about health care. More recently, these countries have shifted their focus to defining a fair process for limit setting and away from searching for general distributive principles (Holm, 2000). This is not to say that general principles offer no guidance—they do—but there remains reasonable disagreement about what guidance they give for real-world decision-making.

In the absence of a broadly accepted consensus on principles for fair distribution, the problem of fair allocation becomes one of procedural justice. The basic idea behind this appeal to procedural justice is quite familiar. When we lack consensus on principles that tell us what is fair, or even when we have general principles but are burdened by reasonable disagreements about how they apply, we may nevertheless find a process or procedure that most can accept as fair to those who are affected by such decisions. That fair process then determines for us what counts as a fair outcome.

Of course, much more needs to be said about what makes a decision process about limits fair to those affected by it. Disagreements about health care resource allocation—such as how much priority to give to the sickest patients—ultimately rest on moral perspectives. We will argue that, because health care limit setting inevitably raises moral controversies, for a decision-making process to be and be seen as fair, it must foster thorough deliberation about the facts, reasons, and principles that are relevant to the dispute. Furthermore, since these limits affect well-being and even liberty in fundamental ways, the reasons that play a role in setting them must be ones that participants can accept as relevant to the decisions (Daniels & Sabin, 1997). This requirement that the grounds for limits be justifiable to all affected by them is an idea well-rooted in the social contract tradition of political philosophy. Ultimately, we shall argue, it means that fair process must enable public deliberation and democratic oversight for health care limits.

Our approach in this book is to recast the problem of limit setting as a question about how decisions about limits should be made. Specifically, *under what conditions should society grant authority to individuals or institutions to set limits to health care?* Under what conditions should people put their lives in the hands of others in this way and give legitimacy to the authority they exercise? This *legitimacy problem,* we believe, is a fundamental problem of ethics and health policy for the 21st century, and it is fundamental, regardless of the details of the financing and delivery systems that differentiate health care systems in different countries.

AN INTERNATIONAL PERSPECTIVE
ON THE LEGITIMACY PROBLEM

Although we believe that every health system must address the problem of legitimacy, public understanding of this problem is dramatically shaped by the different experiences people have of health care delivery in different countries. These differences allow us to locate countries on a social learning curve concerning resource limits and how to manage them fairly. Americans have learned different things from the experience of their health care system than Canadians and Europeans have learned from theirs. The proposals we later offer about how to address the legitimacy problem are ultimately an attempt to help all societies move along that learning curve, regardless of where they now are.

It might seem, however, that we have misidentified the issue. Complaints about the health care system are rarely formulated in terms of legitimacy, whether in the United States or elsewhere. In the United States, people complain about increasing distrust of insurers and doctors, as well as about loss of choice, which they blame on managed care. In many national health insurance or service systems, the complaints are often about underfunding and bureaucratic insensitivity to patient needs. Where does the problem of legitimacy fit in all this?

Loss of trust, diminished choices, underfunding, and bureaucratic insensitivity are all real problems. We believe, however, that these phenomena ultimately rest on the legitimacy problem and cannot be fully addressed unless the legitimacy problem is addressed as well. To show this, we need to consider the social context in these different settings more carefully.

People in countries like Sweden, Norway, the Netherlands, Germany, Great Britain, and Canada, among others, have had two to three generations of experience with their national health insurance or national health service systems. As a result, there is widespread understanding and acceptance of the need to share limited resources under politically negotiated budget constraints. Similarly, there is familiarity with the need for appropriate institutional authorities, empowered by the political process, to make decisions that affect access to medical services. People in these countries are more aware than are Americans that these decisions limit the choices available to physicians and patients—especially since they will have had to queue for some procedures, even as the media and the Internet make them more aware of new treatments. Public awareness has, however, been shaped by decades of experience of sharing resources to meet population needs, not the revolutionary transformation experienced more recently by Americans.

In countries with universal coverage systems, awareness of legitimacy is focused less on *who* exercises authority and more on *how* that authority should be exercised. Are limit-setting decisions bureaucratically arbitrary? Are they made in response to clamor about budgets that is insensitive to the actual needs of critically ill patients? Are the decisions transparent, so that people affected by them know why they are made? Is there a way to appeal these decisions and to promote further deliberation about them?

These questions about *how* to set limits have precipitated a broad debate about the relative merits of *explicit* and *implicit* rationing. Explicit approaches create public criteria for setting priorities and openly acknowledge the limits these criteria entail; implicit approaches ask authorities to apply pragmatic forms of "muddling through," largely behind the scenes (Klein, 1995; Klein, Day & Redmayne, 1996; Mechanic, 1997a; Smith, 1991). Throughout this book, we develop a "middleway" position that seeks to incorporate the strengths and insights of both the explicit and implicit approaches to limit setting.

The questions about *how* to make limit-setting decisions form the true core of the legitimacy problem. They rapidly rise into public awareness whenever the media capture public attention with a dramatic denial of treatment. For example, when the Cambridge and Huntington Health Authority in England refused funding for a second bone marrow transplant to Jaymee Bowen (known as Child B during the controversy), issues of trust in bureaucratic authorities, fair process, and public accountability for decision-making emerged stage-center (Ham & Pickard, 1998). The same issues have been central in similar cases in Norway, New Zealand, and elsewhere (Coulter & Ham, 2000). The way even reasonable decisions are made and defended to those affected by them determines whether the political system ultimately responsible for limits can implement and stand by them. Despite generations of experience in these systems with meeting population health needs under publicly imposed resource limits, much more social learning still needs to take place about the conditions that sustain legitimacy and trust (Klein, Day & Redmund, 1996).

The experience with limits in the United States is very different. Where countries with national health insurance or services ask *how* to set limits fairly, Americans ask *whether* limits are actually necessary and, if they are, *who* should set them. In the 1990s, millions of Americans suddenly became aware that when they are ill, neither they nor their physicians may have the authority they traditionally had to make crucial decisions about their own treatment. (Many physicians had begun to sense a shift in authority when they encountered revised Medicare reimbursement policies that limited hospital stays in 1983.) Unlike the earlier era of "unmanaged" insurance, at present, considerable authority rests with health plans and, more indirectly, with large employers. Although this fundamental shift in authority raises a clear question about legitimacy, Americans tend to perceive the problem as loss of choice and intrusion by managed care. The most common reaction is diminished trust in physicians and in the system (Mechanic & Schlesinger, 1996; Blendon, Brodie, Benson et al., 1998; Davies, 1999). Not surprisingly, commentators on the American health care system predict the emergence of more consumer driven approaches (Center for Studying Health System Change, 2001) and even "the end of managed care" (Robinson, 2001).

Americans do not interpret changes associated with managed care as a legitimacy problem for a straightforward reason. As a people, Americans do not yet acknowledge the reality of limits in health care. They see no connection between talk about rising costs and any problem of scarcity. Insured Americans, after all, have had decades of experience of medical benefits flowing without constraint and costs rising without visible consequences. Unlike Europeans and Canadians, they do not see the political effects of their demand for health care show up in public debates about national budgets.

It is often said that, "Americans are different," meaning that they are culturally more individualistic than Europeans. This American characteristic is then invoked to explain the emergence of the much more modest social safety net in the United States than in Europe or Canada. But the causal connections between culture and institutions work in both directions. American institutions teach lessons that disguise the need to face limits on resources and to share them fairly, and these messages shape cultural attitudes.

As a result of such experiences over many decades, the American public is much more likely—and with reason—to believe that when employers or health plans are intent on reducing costs, it is because they are primarily thinking about their own "bottom line" or profits. The savings that cost containment aims at— whether through practice guidelines (modes of practice recommended as effective and efficient), utilization management (review of whether the treatment a physician prescribes is truly "necessary"), or new incentive structures to physicians and hospitals (especially systems that put providers at risk for the cost of care)—are seen as reducing patient care in order to increase earnings for employers and health plans. Cost containment is not seen as improving the value for one's money that everyone, purchaser and patient alike, gets in a cooperative venture. It is indeed reasonable for the public to see the savings as *not* mutually beneficial because there is no assurance that savings are redirected to meet the more urgent health care needs of the covered population (Daniels, 1986).

The nation's poor awareness of the underlying problems of scarcity and legitimacy is a result of the way public debate about limit setting has been conducted— or more accurately, not conducted. For Americans, the problem of scarcity and its fair management has not been raised nationally by political leaders in serious debate about public policy, with the notable exception of Oregon's quite public prioritization and rationing of Medicaid services in the early 1990s, to which we return shortly. Instead, the public message for over two decades can be captured in these statements:

- Rapidly rising health care costs, attributed primarily to waste and inefficiency, constitute a crisis for the system.
- America cannot afford to provide everyone with insurance coverage until costs are controlled.
- U.S. business is at a competitive disadvantage worldwide if employers and the government do not rein in these costs.
- The solution is to rely on the efficiency produced by market competition among health providers to drive out waste and lower costs.
- The result will be that we can then afford universal insurance coverage and we will not have to set limits at all.

This public message was explicit even within the national effort at health care reform early in the Clinton administration. In the spring of 1993, the Ethics Working group of Clinton's Health Care Task Force (of which one of us was a member) urged the leadership of the Task Force to address the problem of rationing medical services straightforwardly. The group felt it was crucial to create an ethical framework for rationing since the Administration plan called for charging a national advisory board with the task of updating a benefit package as new technologies emerged (Daniels, 1998a; Brock & Daniels, 1994). That task could involve making choices among beneficial services under resource constraints.

The ethics group was told that the term *rationing* must not be used in any documents or memos produced by it or by the task force. When ethics group members persisted in wanting to discuss the issue, they were granted a special meeting with Ira Magaziner, the administrative manager of the task force, who was directly accountable to Hillary Clinton. After hearing the ethics group's arguments, Magaziner insisted that resources now consumed by unnecessary services would be freed up by the competitive forces the system would unleash and that the rationing of beneficial services would prove unnecessary. Though members of the ethics group agreed that eliminating inefficiency should precede the rationing of beneficial services, it was also clear that the Administration position turned on the political judgment that talk about rationing would scare the public and undermine reform. Ducking the issue did not help, however, since opponents of the plan charged it with rationing, anyway. Indeed, one scurrilous magazine attack that accused the plan of rationing precipitated its completely unknown author into election as lieutenant governor of New York in 1994.

Ironically, with the failure of national insurance reform, it was not "big government," the focus of the expensive "Harry and Louise" advertisements sponsored by health insurers opposed to reform, that took away choices and rationed care. Rather, it was "big business," which was determined to reduce the rate of cost increases it faced in employee benefits. The role of large employers remained largely invisible to the public. Instead of the public blaming employers for the changes they encountered in the system, blame was deflected, with the help of the media, onto managed care companies, the vehicles chosen by big business. Government strategy also came to focus on using managed care to reduce costs in the provision of Medicaid, and later Medicare, services.

In 1995, after the failure of political reform and in the midst of the rapid, market-driven transformation of the U.S. system, we began a study of how managed care organizations make decisions about adding coverage for new technologies. Somewhat naively, we expected that managed care organizations would operate on a budget that would constrain coverage for new services. Such a budget would require comparative decisions in which new technologies, affecting different groups of patients with different conditions, would compete with each other for scarce resources. Our project, we hoped, would reveal the visible tip of the rationing iceberg.

To our surprise, we found no comparative decision-making under budgets in the coverage decisions for new technologies, despite the intense competitive climate forced by large employers bidding down premiums. Committees deliberating about coverage of new technologies gave no explicit consideration to the "opportunity cost" of these decisions (Daniels & Sabin, 1998a). Even pharmacy committees, which often make coverage decisions that involve comparing several drugs, are making decisions only within drug categories, not across categories that meet quite different health needs.

When we asked medical directors and other key administrators why technology assessment was carried out without such budget constraints, we received two answers. First, the medical directors claimed there were still other ways to save resources, and so imposing a budget and forcing comparative decisions among safe and efficacious services was not yet necessary. Second, they believed that comparative decisions were a form of explicit rationing that should be governed by societal decisions and directives, not by the decisions of private organizations. Here the medical directors were sensitive to the legitimacy problem. They also expressed fear of being identified in the media as an organization that "rationed" care, a label that could have dire market consequences.

The point is that neither the U.S. government nor the private sector (with the exception of the state of Oregon) has been willing to take the heat involved in leading public deliberation about resource limits, the need for setting priorities, and the need for limiting services. Both politicians and corporate managers have a career interest in being seen as giving more, not less, to their constituents, employees, and customers. Of course, American society accepts, and both the government and private insurers carry out, the explicit rationing of care by ability to pay, excluding 45 million people from insurance coverage, even as people litigate and legislate against any exclusion from coverage of even unproven treatments. And all parties—politicians, corporate leaders, and the public—know that current strategies for containing costs *do* limit medical services, whether reasonably or not.

The state of Oregon remains the exception to this sad tale. In the late 1980s, then State Senate President (and later Governor) John Kitzhaber led a campaign to establish reasonable priorities among services provided by Medicaid. Initially, a decision was made not to fund expensive bone marrow transplants for some patients in order to make resources available for prenatal maternal care programs in the state. Coby Howard, a young boy denied such a transplant, became a visible, identified "victim" of the rationing policy when he went on television to raise money for treatment. (In fact, he was actually medically ineligible for the procedure because he was not in remission from his cancer, but the press ignored this issue). National and international attention was focused on the denial.

Quite bravely, Kitzhaber and other Oregon leaders then began a comprehensive public process to establish priorities among Medicaid services. Crucial to the process was the effort to incorporate public values through town meetings, phone surveys, and public hearings. State commissioners charged with setting priorities initially attempted to use cost-effectiveness rankings, but these rankings proved publicly unacceptable, even ludicrous. The commissioners then adopted alternative methods, showing responsiveness to public input and values. Oregon's effort remains a singular experiment internationally because of its effort at transparency through the public justification of rankings and priorities (Kitzhaber, 1993).

We should by no means limit discussion of legitimacy to developed countries and their wealthy health care systems. In developing countries, the legitimacy problem is more urgent and dramatic since scarcity requires more painful choices and much more draconian measures. In many such settings, however, public authorities are widely perceived to be untrustworthy and riddled with corruption. Moreover, the large informal sectors that exist in these economies mean that public resources, raised through taxes, are especially limited. To overcome these public sector limitations, reformers, often pushed by external forces, such as the World Bank, have encouraged the emergence of a large private sector. In theory, the private sector will bring new resources and new efficiencies to the system. In reality, the private sector remains unregulated, is itself riddled with corruption, and often competes with and undermines the public sector. Health reform in these settings must face the legitimacy problem squarely.

In what follows, we focus on solving the legitimacy problem and only secondarily, or derivatively, on specific measures that might be used to increase public trust or decrease distrust. This is not to deny in any way the importance of trust. Still, trust and legitimacy are distinct issues, and both must be addressed. People can trust illegitimate authorities. They also sometimes distrust legitimate ones. If the exercise of legitimate authority generates regular distrust, however, we have reason to question whether the authority is exercised in a truly legitimate manner. We must not only ask, "Can we trust individuals or institutions who benefit by deciding to treat us less or in less costly ways?" We must also ask, "Should we so trust them with the authority to make such decisions?"

ACCOUNTABILITY FOR REASONABLENESS AND THE ARGUMENT OF THIS BOOK

Justice requires limits to care, and the lack of consensus on principles of distribution means that we must develop an acceptable fair process for setting limits and learn how to apply that process in real-world situations. These two claims, sketched briefly above, are developed further in Chapters 2 and 3. In Chapter 4 we argue for four conditions that are necessary if such a process is to address the legitimacy problem. Meeting these conditions makes decision makers "accountable for the reasonableness" of their decisions.

In Chapters 5–9, we illustrate how accountability for reasonableness can be applied in action by drawing on some examples of best practices that emerge from an ongoing series of studies we have conducted of managed care organizations.

Specifically, in Chapter 5, we examine several ways of managing "last chance" experimental therapies, which have often been the focus of litigation and legislative mandates. In Chapter 6, we argue that accountability for reasonableness is necessary given the variation we will inevitably encounter in coverage decisions for such new technologies as lung volume reduction surgery. We consider (in Chapter 7) what implementing accountability for reasonableness would mean in pharmacy benefit management. In Chapter 8, we consider how accountability for reasonableness can be applied when we transfer responsibility for setting limits to physicians, through various economic incentive or reimbursement schemes. We then look, in Chapter 9, at how public contracting for mental health care that is delivered by private, for-profit, managed care organizations can contain measures to ensure such accountability. Taken together, Chapters 5–9 begin to flesh out how society can learn to apply a "middle way" to limit setting that incorporates the strengths and insights of both the implicit and explicit rationing approaches. Our goal in these chapters is to show in a practical way how institutions can be shaped to make them more accountable for reasonableness. What emerges, however, is not a set of rules or an algorithm that can deliver specific answers about what limits are fair in specific cases. The whole argument of this book is that we lack consensus on such rules and must, instead, rely on fair deliberative procedures that yield a range of acceptable answers. We believe this accountability for reasonableness is a requirement for the legitimacy of any system that sets limits, including European systems of universal coverage, the current American managed care format and the consumer choice models being predicted as the next step for the United States (Center for Studying Health System Change, 2001; Robinson, 2001).

In Chapter 10 we return to a theme already prominent in this chapter—that the legitimacy problem is international and affects health care systems at all levels of development and with various methods of financing and organization. Specifically, we look at how "accountability for reasonableness" has become the focus, in content if not in name, of concerns about the decision-making process in several universal-coverage systems. We also briefly explore its relevance to health care reform in developing countries.

We conclude with a discussion of the social learning curve that was referred to earlier. Our approach to the legitimacy problem is a long-term one, setting conditions under which public understanding of limits and deliberation about them can be improved and suggesting how these conditions can be applied in real-world action. The focus on social learning, and its relevance to deliberative process and democratic control, will be more apparent if we describe, however briefly, the notion of "accountability for reasonableness."

We propose four conditions that are necessary if a decision-making process about health care limits is to address the legitimacy problem (Daniels & Sabin, 1997). First, limit-setting decisions must be public. Not only must the decisions themselves be public, but the grounds for making them must be public as well.

This *Publicity Condition* ensures transparency. Notice that it does not require that all criteria for decision-making be set in advance or explicitly agreed upon ahead of time. There is room for appropriate authorities and institutions to develop such criteria as they face problems over time. The transparency condition establishes, however, the potential for developing a robust kind of "case law" regarding limit-setting decisions.

Second, the grounds for decisions must be ones that fair-minded people can agree are relevant to meeting health care needs fairly under reasonable resource constraints. This *Relevancy Condition* is crucial because it focuses deliberation about limits on a shared goal, or common good. Some kinds of reasons are easier to get agreement on than others: safety and efficacy, for example, will be less problematic, by themselves, than cost-effectiveness. The methodology of cost-effectiveness may carry with it some distributive assumptions that have to be explicitly addressed and agreed upon before they can meet the Relevancy Condition. In the American system and in many systems in developing countries, a private, for-profit sector raises important questions about the kinds of reasons stakeholders can perceive as relevant and what kinds of information would be needed to establish that relevance.

Third, limit-setting decisions must be subject to *revision and appeal,* and the process for doing that must itself meet the first two conditions. More generally, decisions must be revisable over time in light of better evidence, arguments, and deliberation. Finally, there must be some form of *regulation* to ensure that the other conditions are met.

The approach we sketch here and develop later is ultimately aimed at enhancing control over limit-setting decisions and the public deliberation that is so central to a democracy. Regardless of the details of the design of a health care system—whether it is a public health service, as in the United Kingdom or Norway, a national health insurance scheme with a single payer, as in Canada, with multiple payers, as in Germany and the Netherlands, or a mixed public and private system without true universal coverage, as in the United States and many developing countries—legitimate authority ultimately rests in the control that democratic process exercises over the system. We think our account of fair process enhances the public learning that is needed to empower the public to exercise appropriate democratic control over health care.

2

JUSTICE, SCARCITY, AND PUBLIC ACCOUNTABILITY FOR LIMITS

Justice, we stipulated in Chapter 1, requires meeting health care needs fairly under resource constraints, and this, in turn, requires limiting care in a publicly accountable way. We were trying to be succinct, not glib. Yet glib we might seem. The notions we appeal to—justice, meeting needs fairly, and public accountability—may seem like "apple pie and motherhood," but they are all controversial. Critics may see them as naive and abstract. How could ideas like these possibly have relevance for hands-on health practice?

Justice, the Health-Is-Priceless Advocate insists, requires that we treat medical needs as more important than nearly any of the other things on which we spend our money. What could be more important than extending healthy lives by curing or preventing disease or disability? For Health-Is-Priceless Advocates, justice means meeting medical needs regardless of what seems to compete with them.

The Scarcity Skeptic insists there is no true scarcity, only waste, or irrationality, or the frivolity of trivial pursuits. There is no real scarcity when billions are spent on unnecessary tests and procedures, or highly paid health care executives, or dividends to investors. If there were true scarcity, individuals would not spend their money on face lifts and hair transplants, unproven "alternative" treatments, or expensive "natural" diet supplements. If there were true scarcity, society would not invest in new antimissile systems or tax breaks for the very rich. Scarcity Skeptics think scarcity is scare talk that diverts us from the need to seek efficiency.

For the Market Hawk, we appeared glib when we asserted that justice means that we owe each other robust systems of medical care. All we really owe each other, the Market Hawks insist, are efficient insurance schemes and the choice, with good information, to buy or leave them as we prefer. Maybe—just maybe— we owe the very poor a decent, limited, minimum of care, but that does not mean we all face a general problem of limits to care. Of course, it is childish to deny that there is scarcity, but scarcity does not require someone imposing limits on our care. Properly functioning markets for health care or medical insurance put prices on what we want. Prices reflect supply and demand. If some kinds of health care cost more than we are willing to pay, we limit ourselves by not buying it. *That* is all Market Hawks think we need by way of accountability.

The Implicit Rationer agrees that justice requires limits to care but rejects our assertion that public accountability is required in setting limits as unrealistic. Human nature is inherently self-centered. However much lip service we may give to fairness, when push comes to shove, we will advocate for ourselves and our loved ones. Although we may favor equitable resource allocation in principle, we will inevitably favor coverage for the diseases we and those whom we care most about have suffered from. It is much better, Implicit Rationers claim, to leave the task to experts who are free to "muddle through" behind the scenes and actually deliver reasonable distributions. Opening the whole process to public scrutiny will only encourage litigation and special lobbying of politicians and public officials. Juries cannot resist pillaging deep pockets, and public officials cannot say no to constituents. Explicitness may be desirable in theory, but it creates more tension than social systems can tolerate. Better quiet, if imperfect, justice than the agitation and instability created by public accountability (Calabresi & Bobbitt, 1978).

Clearly, we owe the reader a defense of our earlier assertions against these criticisms. In this chapter we respond primarily to the Health-is-Priceless Advocate and the Scarcity Skeptic, explaining why we think that, although health care is of special moral importance, finite resources mean we must, nevertheless, place limits on care. Not only our preferred account of justice but a broader family of views about justice has similar implications for limit setting. Our remarks about justice and the special moral importance of health care are also part of our reply to the Market Hawk. In the next chapter we further reply to the Market Hawk, but especially to the Implicit Rationer by showing why we cannot establish the legitimacy and fairness of limits without public accountability and fair procedures for setting them.

THE SPECIAL MORAL IMPORTANCE OF HEALTH CARE

In nearly all societies, people believe that access to health care should be based on need, not on ability to pay. In many, if not most, cases, they not only believe this but act on their beliefs. Whatever other, often vast, inequalities are tolerated, health care is distributed much more equitably. Thus, all advanced industrialized societies other than the United States, and some developing countries as well, have universal-coverage health systems or medical insurance. Even the United States, which tolerates enormous inequalities in income and wealth, provides means-tested insurance for the very poor and universal coverage for the elderly and people with serious disabilities.

What justifies the view that health care is of special moral importance in this way?

A common first response is to suggest that health care is of special moral importance because it is a necessary condition for happiness. This response overstates the point. People can be happy despite being ill or disabled.[1] Nevertheless, the tendency of disease and disability to undermine happiness or welfare gives special reason for utilitarians to support providing universal access to needed medical services as one important way of promoting aggregate welfare. This way of answering the question about the specialness of health care leaves plenty of room—some might complain *too much* room—for other ways of promoting aggregate welfare to compete with health care. As a result, the utilitarian argument concludes that people owe each other only that level of health care that promotes aggregate welfare.[2]

The specialness of health care is better understood in a different way—for which one of us has argued in detail elsewhere (Daniels, 1985). Rather than rely on the tendency of disease and disability to interfere with happiness, we emphasize the way in which these adverse departures from normal functioning[3] reduce the range of opportunities people would otherwise enjoy. The central moral importance, for purposes of justice, of preventing and treating disease and disability with effective health care services (construed broadly to include public health and environmental measures, as well as personal medical services) derives from the way in which protecting normal functioning contributes to protecting opportunity. Specifically, by keeping people close to normal functioning, health care preserves the capabilities individuals need to participate in the political, social, and economic life of their society. It sustains them as fully participating citizens—normal collaborators and competitors—in all spheres of social life.

This relationship between health care and the protection of opportunity suggests that the appropriate principle of distributive justice for regulating the design of a health care system is a robust principle protecting available opportunities. Historically, however, we have thought about the protection of equal opportunity more narrowly. In American civil rights legislation, for example, we protect equal opportunity, understood as "careers open to talents," when we make sure jobs and offices are open to all solely on the basis of their talents and skills. Society prohibits barriers, legal or customary, based on irrelevant traits of individuals, such as race, gender, or social class.

In practice, however, many people believe that we violate the spirit of this narrow, or formal, principle of equal opportunity when we allow unfair social practices, such as race, gender, or class bias, or the morally arbitrary contingencies of birth into one social class rather than another, to lead to the underdevelopment of talents, skills, and capabilities. Not correcting for these effects of race, gender, or class means that people cannot compete in a fair way for jobs and offices and the rewards that attend them—even if we formally prohibit discrimination. In recent political philosophy, John Rawls (1971), therefore, advocates a more robust principle he calls "fair equality of opportunity." This stronger principle requires that we design institutions, such as public education and early childhood programs, including child care, that help correct for the influence of race, gender, and class in societies where such divisions have historically played an important role in shaping opportunity.

Applying the fair-equality-of-opportunity principle to health care carries us one step further. We must now think of disease and disability as creating additional obstacles that we have obligations to eliminate in order for us to have "fair opportunities." Though this extension of the fair opportunity principle would explain and justify our felt obligations to assist each other in meeting medical needs, and thus answer the question about the special importance of health care, it faces two objections worth discussing.

One objection is that, historically, we think of protecting opportunity against social contingencies, such as socioeconomic inequalities or other inequalities in the treatment of races, ethnic groups, religions, genders, or classes. Traditionally, we think we are giving people equal opportunity if we allow them to compete fairly for jobs and offices on the basis of "relevant traits," even though these talents and skills differ as a result of the "natural lottery" for biological differences that we all think normal. Since we typically think of disease and disability as the result of natural processes, that is, as chance or a natural lottery, we should not appeal to a principle protecting opportunity to address medical needs. People who think of disease or disability as unfortunate but not unfair would accordingly strongly resist this extension of the fair equality of opportunity principle.

Although we may typically think of disease and disability as the result of chance, not social factors, in doing so, we miss an important fact. Without denying that much disease and disability is the result of a natural lottery, the incidence and distribution of disease and disability is heavily influenced by such non-health-care determinants as levels of income, education, socioeconomic inequality, political participation, investment in social capital, and cultural and religious practices (Daniels, Kennedy & Kawachi, 1999, 2000; Kawachi, Kennedy & Wilkinson, 1999). It is more difficult than we might think to separate the influence of social practices from natural events. Consequently, stretching the fair-equality-of-opportunity principle so that it applies to health and health care crosses a line that is less clear than it might seem at first. In any case, in crossing that line, we capture the widely held belief—ignored by those who say disease or disability are unfortunate but not unfair—that we owe assistance to each other to correct for the contingencies of disease and disability.

Expanding the fair-equality-of-opportunity principle to include the effects of disease and disability raises a different, philosophically more interesting, objection as well. Once we decide to protect opportunities by correcting for such effects of the natural lottery as disease and disability, then consistency seems to require that we also correct for other effects of the natural lottery. Why stop with disease or disability? Our talents and skills themselves are also affected by our genes and other biological factors in development. They are the product of both a natural and social lottery. As a result, a principle protecting equality of opportunity, or one giving priority to reducing deficits in opportunity, should require that society correct for all naturally, as well as socially, imposed disadvantages, not just those that occur when we lose normal functioning. It requires leveling the playing field more dramatically to include all the ways our talents and skills might put us at a disadvantage relative to others.[4] So extended, it protects us against cosmic bad luck.

For both theoretical and policy reasons, we have argued elsewhere that it is plausible to draw the line roughly where we do, focusing on the way normal functioning protects fair opportunity and resisting the radical extension of the appeal to equal opportunity.[5] The primary rationale for health care in our view focuses on correcting for the impact of disease and disability, not for enhancing otherwise normal but disadvantageous traits. Our intention here, however, is to emphasize a shared feature of these different ways of appealing to the connection between opportunities and health or health care. It is what these views share, rather than how they differ, that is central to the argument of this book. An account of distributive justice that strengthens the opportunity principle even further than we do, so that it corrects for more aspects of natural bad luck than simply meeting medical needs, or that focuses on assuring people of the capabilities, or "positive freedom," they need to function as free and equal citizens, as Amartya Sen proposes, still has the implications that concern us in this book.[6]

Our account shares with the stronger opportunity principle and other egalitarian views two key features. First, health care is of special moral importance because of its central (if limited) contribution to protecting our opportunities or capabilities. Our social obligations to protect opportunity—our rights to equal opportunity—give us claims on others for appropriate forms of health care. A right to health care is thus a special case of a right to equal opportunity.[7]

A second shared feature is the fact that society has to set limits to health care, despite its special moral importance. Together, these shared features of the opportunity-based approaches support an obligation to provide appropriate medical services on the basis of need, not ability to pay, subject to reasonable resource constraints. It thus provides an ethical justification for universal coverage health services or insurance schemes. It also suggests that we judge the importance of health care needs by their impact on opportunity and take some guidance from this idea in setting limits to care. Our entitlements to health care will thus be relative to many judgments made about the appropriate services to provide given levels of knowledge and resources available in the society. Despite these shared features, the family of views of justice will differ about some specifics. There will be differences, for example, about how much inequality, or "tiering," is permitted, or about just what kinds of rationing are implied (e.g., a focus on treatment, not enhancement; rationing by age). Nevertheless, it is their shared features that primarily occupy us in what follows.

IF HEALTH CARE IS SPECIAL, WHY IMPOSE LIMITS?

Health care competes with other goods.   It may seem paradoxical that an account that builds centrally on the intuition that health care is so special carries with it the implication that we must set limits to it. This appearance of paradox is an illusion, and in dispelling the illusion, we reply to the Health-Is-Priceless Advocate.

Though health care is important to the protection of opportunity, it is not the only good that is important in this way. As important as it is, it is by no means the only important social good. Limits arise from both these facts.

Many things affect and protect opportunities. Education, job training, job creation—even law and order—contribute to protecting our opportunities and to supporting our relevant capabilities. We must make reasonable decisions about how to support all these and other opportunity-promoting measures with the resources we have.

Opportunity is not the only important social good. Basic liberties must be protected. This protection means supporting institutions that defend people against the violation of those liberties, but it also means that we require investments in institutions that assure our citizens that they can effectively exercise their liberties, especially their rights of political participation.

Opportunity is expanded as we increase societal wealth and knowledge. But expanding the social pie may require introducing incentives that encourage some inequalities. To the extent that economic growth is improved by permitting some inequalities, even if we only allow inequalities that help those who are worst off (Rawls, 1971), we create a tension between equality of opportunity and expansion of opportunities. In addition, the literature on the social determinants of health suggests that social and economic inequalities, and not just the deprivation of the very poor, produce inequalities in health (and thus in opportunity). As a result, decisions about economic growth rates and social policies that affect them are inextricably connected to decisions that affect the levels of health needs and the resources available to meet them.

In short, however important health care is, we must weigh it against other goods and other ways of promoting opportunity. Investing in health care has "opportunity costs" even though it contributes to promoting opportunity. The Health-Is-Priceless Advocate has too simple a picture of the world of value.

How we decide about health care vs. other goods matters, but however we decide, the limits to resources are real.   Many publicly financed health care systems operate under global budgets, whether these systems are organized as a national health service or a national insurance system, and whether or not they are financed by general tax revenues, payroll taxes, or (mandatory) insurance premiums. In setting these global budgets, public officials and the political process weigh investment in health care against other investments that support different social goods. They must consider how much to invest in education or child care, or pension funds and unemployment benefits, or tax incentives to industry or military defense and police. This public trade-off process sets limits to care.

If we examine different systems, we see that they fund health services at quite different levels. Some universal-coverage systems with good health outcomes budget only 5% or 6% of gross domestic product on health care. Others budget 8% to 10%. The United States spends over 14%. These differences reflect various facts about these different societies, including the organization of the health sector and how efficient it is, as well as the society's demographics and its cultural and political characteristics.

From these variations in choices about levels of health expenditure, we might conclude that there is no one reasonable or fair level of investment in health, no magic number that is the fair allocation to health care. Alternatively, we might conclude that what is reasonable and fair for a society is highly dependent on the context. The salient point is that, in some countries, these variations emerge from a political process that involves public deliberation about resource constraints.

By way of contrast, in the United States and other mixed public and private systems, there is nothing resembling a global budget, and there is no mechanism for setting limits to health-sector resources through a democratic political process. Instead, some parts of the system are governed by public-sector decisions, while other limits are set by private organizations and the aggregate effect of many individual decisions. Key among the private decision makers in America are the employers who receive tax benefits for providing medical insurance. Where present, unions that negotiate the level of employee health benefits also shape health care allocation. It has been large employers who have played a leading role in setting resource limits that have driven the cost-containment efforts in the American health sector.

In such a mixed system, it is clearly much more difficult to set resource limits in a reasonable way that is based on societal deliberation about the relative importance of competing goods. Because the key elements are never on the same table at the same time, the different sectors and interests end up setting limits for largely local reasons. As a result, it is much easier in the United States to conclude that efforts to set limits or contain costs are the result of self-interest, not guided by any consideration of how to achieve the common good.

Nevertheless, if a political system delegates, if only by default, the responsibility for setting limits to private agents, such as employers, who are not accountable to their workers the way that elected representatives are accountable to the electorate, then that system is stuck with the results of choices made by those private agents. The fact that limits are not set in an ideal way is not a justification for concluding or pretending that they do not exist or are not real constraints. If people do not like the resource limits or the way they were set, they have to change the system, but even if they do, they will end up with some other set of limits.

Our argument in what follows takes the inevitability of limits as a given—though we readily admit that a more just system might indeed have more reasonable limits set through a different and more accountable process. But the fact that the United States ought to seek more reasonable overall resource limits does not imply that we need not develop a fair, publicly accountable process for allocating the resources that are available.

The point is simple: One injustice does not excuse another.

Inefficiency interferes with meeting needs fairly, but we cannot avoid trying to set limits fairly just because we encounter inefficiency. People who deny scarcity often focus on waste and inefficiency. The Scarcity Skeptic has a valid point, but we should not let it turn into an evasion of responsibility. The valid point is this: Whatever overall resources are available for health care, if they are inefficiently and ineffectively used, then fewer needs will be met. People will be able to make the legitimate complaint that they are being denied care that a more efficient—but not richer—system would have given them. Their complaint is that they are being made to pay the price of inefficiency (Himmelstein & Woolhandler, 1986). And they are right.

This objection only shows, however, that we should work hard to make systems more efficient. Doing so will contribute to the fairness of the system overall (see Daniels, Light & Caplan, 1996; Daniels, Bryant, Castano et al., 2000). It does not mean, however, that we should evade an effort to allocate what is left as a result of inefficiency in a fair, publicly accountable way.

Part of the reason the Scarcity Skeptic's valid point sometimes slides into an evasion is that we generally believe that inefficiency is always avoidable and is the result of various things we can all agree are bad. But some inefficiency, especially in the medical context, may well be unavoidable. In a classic discussion of medical markets, Nobel Laureate Kenneth Arrow (1963) traced many forms of inefficiency and market aberration to the presence of high levels of uncertainty. Doctors are often uncertain what condition a patient has, and they are often uncertain what interventions are most likely to be effective. Patients face even greater degrees of uncertainty. Where there is considerable uncertainty, it is common to find great variation in the decisions physicians and patients make about treatment. Evidence suggests that this variation does not reflect differences in the incidence of disease and that higher levels of treatment do not produce better outcomes. We then look at the variation and conclude that much of the utilization we see is unnecessary and therefore avoidable.

Some of that variation, however, is the result of different attitudes toward risk taking and the value of using marginally better treatments. Whereas some doctors and patients might be persuaded by an appeal that they abide by the dictates of "evidence-based medicine" or expert decisions about "practice guidelines," others, especially given the uncertainty, may think it worth the investment of resources to go the extra mile in aggressive treatment. Different values are at work, and they contribute to what we typically see as inefficiency. Inefficiency can be the result of choice, not simply of stupidity.

Whether it is values that contribute to inefficiency, or only the uncertainty that gives more room for those values to enter the picture, the result is that we may have a considerable degree of inefficiency that we cannot eliminate simply by appealing to rationality. The ideal of "medical enlightenment" will only take us so far. If we have to live with some level of inefficiency, then, we had better learn to do so in a way that is fair to all.

The objection from "profits" and the worry that savings do not help those in medical need.   One common reason for refusing to accept the idea of limits is the fact that some health plans, especially for-profit plans, spend as much as 25%–50% of every premium dollar on nonmedical benefits. These dollars go to marketing, administrative costs, and returns to investors. If so much of their premium revenue is drained into costs that deliver no direct benefit to patients, then how can we tolerate the limits these plans set on beneficial services? This complaint has great power and resonates with many practitioners, who believe it gives them an excuse to "game the system" and find ways to benefit patients by breaking or avoiding rules intended to contain costs.

Years ago, one of us argued that, in the American system, it was especially hard to say "no" (or set limits) because savings were not part of a closed system of resource allocation (Daniels, 1986). As a result, practitioners and patients could reasonably worry that savings would not be converted into medical benefits. Doctors might then feel justified in providing the marginal benefit they are trained to deliver rather than relying on a system that might convert savings from constrained modes of practice into profits or into less important benefits elsewhere. Since then, practitioners themselves have been swept into a system of incentives intended to give them a direct stake in reducing the cost of care, which further complicates the moral equation.

It strains credulity to claim that patients can be better served by "efficient" plans that nevertheless drain 25%–30% of every premium dollar away from patient treatment than by nonprofit plans with much lower administrative costs. Yet, it is an article of faith for many Market Hawks in the United States that this is the case. Some people point to the intense competition among plans that temporarily lowered the rate of medical cost increases in the middle of the 1990s as evidence that the faith is justified, but others note that costs began to increase again at the end of the decade and that some of the savings for large purchasers may have been the result of cost shifting to patients and the increasing numbers of uninsured.

We make the same point in response to this critique of profit-driven cost containment that we made earlier about non-ideal resource allocation and inefficiency. One injustice does not justify another. If it can be shown that market competition among for-profit health plans and other medical entrepreneurs works to the disadvantage of patients—as compared to other ways of organizing and delivering care—then we should seek a more just system, one that puts medical dollars to use for their intended purpose. That is clearly a political task—comprehensive reform of the system—and we advocate it.

But that political task is not a substitute for the one we discuss here. Even systems with universal coverage and strong solidarity values face the same problems of limits the United States faces, since the main cost driver over time is the advance of medical technology (see Chapter 10). Avoiding discussion of how to set limits fairly thus risks adding unfair limit setting to a system that is already unfair in other ways.

Though health care has special moral importance, justice still requires that we set limits on its provision. The fact of non-ideal conditions does not exempt us from the task of learning to set limits fairly. The U.S. health care system may be inefficient in various ways; it may drain resources intended for medical benefit away from patients and into the pockets of insurance companies and providers. We should try to correct these problems as best we can, but we should not use the fact that they exist to evade the need to address the long-term problem of setting limits fairly. That is a task we must face regardless of the design of our system, its degree of efficiency, and its method of financing.

In the next chapter, we turn to our earlier claim that setting limits must be done through a fair and publicly accountable process.

NOTES

1. Nor do we obviously owe each other whatever it takes to make us happy. Believing that we do would make us hostage to whatever desires people cultivate (Dworkin, 1981; Rawls, 1982; Daniels, 1985). More plausible is the claim that we owe each other equal opportunity for happiness or advantage (Arneson, 1988; Cohen, 1989), but this view brings us much closer to the position argued for above. For some differences see Daniels, 1996, Ch 10) and Daniels (2002).

2. There is a well-known gap between the view that the right thing to do is to promote aggregate welfare through the universal provision of needed medical services and the claim that it is a requirement of justice that we do so. We leave aside the long-standing philosophical debate about whether this gap is readily closed. Our intention here is only to show that a utilitarian account is compatible with the idea that health care is of special moral importance and yet requires limits. Historically, this should not be surprising since utilitarian reformers have for a century and a half supported various kinds of welfare improvements for the poor and near poor, including universal access to health care.

3. Disease and disability, both physical and mental, are construed as adverse departures from, or impairments of, species-typical normal functional organization, or "normal functioning." The biomedical sciences for humans, like the veterinary sciences for animals, studies both the variation in the functional organization typical for our species and the departures from normal functioning that we call disease and disability (or pathology, more comprehensively) (Boorse, 1975, 1976, 1977, 1997, in press; Daniels 1985). The line between disease and disability and normal functioning is thus drawn in the relatively objective and non-evaluative context provided by the biomedical sciences, broadly construed. What counts as a disease or disability from the perspective of these sciences is largely free from controversy in the broad range of cases. Of course, sometimes, value judgments, including prejudices, as well as errors, intrude, and we get examples of conditions or behaviors that are improperly classified as disease or disability, e.g. the "disease" of masturbation (Engelhardt, 1974) or homosexuality (Bayer, 1981). But just as whales are not fishes, though they were long classified as such, so, too, these conditions are not diseases, even if complex social conditions and attitudes contributed to their being viewed as such.

4. When John Rawls discusses the intuition that the results of both social and natural lotteries are "morally arbitrary," he proposes that we combine the fair-equality-of-opportunity principle, which corrects for social contingencies, with a principle that allows inequalities only if they help to make those who are worst off as well off as possible. This "Difference Principle" mitigates, but does not eliminate, the effects of the natural lottery. Egalitarian proponents of "equal opportunity for welfare or advantage" complain that Rawls's division of labor between his principles fails to correct enough for the moral arbitrariness of natural contingencies. For a defense of Rawls's approach, see Daniels, (2002); see Buchanan, Brock, Daniels & Wikler, (2000) for a discussion of whether our increasing ability to modify the distribution of capabilities through genetic knowledge means justice requires those interventions.

5. The "equal opportunity for advantage" view depends on a troubling distinction between "brute" (or natural) luck and "option" luck, which results from our choices. People have claims on others for assistance when their disadvantages are due to bad brute luck but not bad option luck. If we are interested in protecting our capabilities as citizens, however, we may not want to place such heavy weight on the notion of choice or responsibility for our needs (Anderson, 1999). In addition, people must still be able to agree when someone has deficit in opportunity that gives rise to claims on others: Do we owe each other cosmetic surgery so that we can each have more opportunity to attract mates or dates or modeling jobs? Perhaps the main cases on which we will reach public agreement will be disease and disability, in which case, the view is closer in practice to the view that focuses on protecting normal functioning. There are also administrative and cost problems with this account: Can we really tell just when bad luck is due to choices, or are we dependent on self-reporting? Is what we owe each other too costly to provide? For further discussion, see Daniels, (1996, Ch.10); Sabin & Daniels, (1994); Buchanan, Brock, Daniels & Wikler, (2000); and Daniels (2002).

6. We thus locate our approach within a family of views that, despite their differences, emphasize equal opportunity or that give priority to improving the situation of those with the worst opportunities (see Arneson (1988) and Cohen (1989)). The family also includes Sen's (1992, 1999) much more influential advocacy of a "capability" for "positive freedom" approach to justice. All these views recognize that justice must work under resource limitations, however special the importance of opportunity or freedom.

7. Some recent philosophical literature (cf. Parfit, 1991) has urged that we not talk about strict equality but about giving priority to improving the opportunities (or welfare or well-being or resources) of those with the worst opportunities. On such a prioritarian (as opposed to egalitarian) view, the right to health care would be a special case of the prioritarian right to have opportunity protected.

3

THE LEGITIMACY PROBLEM
AND FAIR PROCESS

Justice requires setting fair limits to health care, but who should set such limits and how? Under what conditions will the limits be seen to be fair and legitimate? In fact, decisions to limit health care are made by many different people at different levels within the health-care system. They have a broad range of consequences, some significant, some barely noticeable, for patients:

- You have scoliosis, a curvature of the spine, and your Canadian primary care physician puts you on the queue for a CT scan. Because he does not rate your condition as highly urgent, you will wait several weeks, perhaps a couple of months, to find out if the condition is causing organ complications.
- You go to the pharmacy to fill a prescription for a new anti-migraine medication that you have seen advertised as the best thing available. You discover that it requires prior approval, and your health plan will pay for the prescription only if you have unsuccessfully tried more traditional, less expensive remedies first.
- Your pulmonologist recommends a new treatment for your advanced emphysema, a surgical procedure that reduces lung volume and has some promising outcomes. Medicare will not cover the procedure unless you are enrolled in a clinical trial in which you may be given an alternative treatment.

25

- Your child's pediatrician, responding to the reimbursement incentives in his capitated practice, decides to prescribe Ritalin to your child to see how it works for him instead of recommending that he receive a more comprehensive neuropsychological workup.
- Your oncologist has persuaded you that an experimental procedure offers your daughter her "last chance" at treatment of her leukemia, but the district health authority (in Great Britain) or your health plan (in the United States) has refused to cover the costs of the treatment.

Despite the range of effects these examples have on patients, they share two important features. First, though all of them may be portrayed as "medical," "technical," or "contractual," they all rest on value judgments about which reasonable people may disagree. For example, some people will give considerable weight to the urgency of the child with leukemia; others will argue that we will not be able to meet other, equally urgent needs if we do not carefully steward resources by excluding unproven treatments. Reasonable people may disagree about how much weight to give to these two factors (see Chapter 5). In several of the other examples, people will disagree about how to value a modest gain in efficacy or reduced side effects if it brings with it a significant increase in costs. Sometimes these limits will provoke open moral and legal controversy. Often, the moral controversy underlying them is resolved quietly and invisibly behind the scenes.

Second, these examples raise questions about fairness and legitimacy that are most appropriately posed from the perspective of those who are denied the care. Thus we should pose the question about legitimacy in this way: Why or when—under what conditions—should a patient or clinician who thinks an uncovered service is appropriate or even "medically necessary" accept as legitimate the limit setting decision of a health plan or district authority? The legitimacy problem asks under what conditions moral authority over these matters should be placed in the hands of private organizations, such as health plans, or even the administrators or panels of experts who make such decisions, and the rules governing them, in public agencies. This is not just a question about *who* makes the decisions, and about whether they have conflicts of interest *when* they make them. It is about *how* they are made. Must legitimate authorities, for example, openly share the reasons for their decisions, or is it enough for them to publicly announce the results of their deliberations?

The question about fairness should also be posed from the perspective of the patient denied care: When does a patient or clinician who thinks an uncovered service appropriate or even "medically necessary" have sufficient reason to accept as fair the limit-setting decisions of a health plan or public authority? Addressing the fairness problem requires consideration of the various reasons that play a role in the decision.

The legitimacy and fairness problems are distinct issues of justice. A legitimate authority can act unfairly, and an illegitimate one can deliver fair decisions. Still, they are related. We may reasonably accept an authority as legitimate only if it abides by a procedure or process or even substantive constraints, such as Constitutional protections, that we consider generally fair. If the authority abandons fair procedure, it may lose its legitimacy. Similarly, in contexts where an authority that claims no legitimacy employs a fair procedure, especially where there may be prior disagreement about what counts as a fair outcome, we may accept the outcome as fair.

In the next chapter, we propose a general solution to the legitimacy and fairness problems. We describe and defend key features of the publicly accountable fair process through which limit-setting decisions should be made. In later chapters, we return to the examples of limit setting mentioned above in some detail: "last chance" therapies, limits on new technologies or pharmacy benefits, and indirect limits influenced by reimbursement methods. Our goal is to illustrate what the fair process we describe looks like when it is applied, for we are proposing a practical, not merely a theoretical, solution to the fairness and legitimacy problems.

Before developing our solution and illustrating it, we take the rest of this chapter to substantiate our claim that we need an account of fair process. Showing that commonly advocated alternative accounts of fairness and legitimacy cannot work, at least when taken by themselves, is central to justifying our account. Specifically, we briefly review and reject four distinct alternatives. The market alternative—we call it "market accountability"—insists that there is no special problem of fairness or legitimacy, provided that we make available a market for insurance in which people legitimize the limits health plans employ by choosing—buying—the plan. Our reply in this chapter to market accountability completes our response to the Market Hawk who spoke up in Chapter 2.

The Implicit Rationer of Chapter 2 might appeal to any of three further alternatives that we describe and respond to here as the basis for his limit-setting policies. The Philosopher's Alternative says that the principles of justice, or some middle-level principles, give us clear enough answers to questions about distributive fairness to determine if fair outcomes are present. The Majority Rule solution suggests that we resolve disputes about limits the way we resolve many policy disputes, through direct or indirect democratic processes that ultimately rely on voting. Since voting is procedurally fair, we should accept the outcome of such voting as fair. The fourth alternative—the Public Attitudes approach—relies not on voting but on scientifically surveying the public to find out its moral views on limits. Using survey results, we can then construct a decision procedure, or technique, that is sensitive to public values about limit setting. Implicit Rationers can use any of these three alternatives—the Philosopher's appeal to principles, the Majority Rule appeal to voting, or the Public Attitude appeal to surveys—to justify their policies. Insofar as these alternatives fail to provide an adequate basis for fairness and legitimacy, however, the Implicit Rationer's argument for behind-the-scenes "muddling through" as a basis for limit setting is weakened.

All these alternatives contain valuable clues to, or elements of, a plausible solution to the legitimacy problem, but taken by themselves, they are inadequate. Because these solutions fail by themselves, we need the account of fair process that we propose in the next chapter. Such a fair process will be enhanced by elements of the other approaches—by the good information about options that market accountability requires, by clear discussion of moral principles and reasons backed by philosophical arguments, by ultimate accountability to societal democratic processes, by contributions from social science about public attitudes and values, and by the Implicit Rationer's understanding of how social systems really work. But without a fair process, none of the other approaches suffices to answer the fairness and legitimacy questions posed by those affected by medical limit setting. We must move beyond the views of the Market Hawk and Implicit Rationer to an account of fair process.

MARKET ACCOUNTABILITY

The central idea behind the market alternative is that there is nothing unfair about limits that we encounter when we make informed purchases of health insurance; indeed, we each legitimize these limits with our purchase of the insurance plan.

The claim that there is no problem of legitimacy or fairness is put forcefully in the following argument, which we shall call the "car purchase analogy." As long as there is clear coverage language in subscriber contracts, there is no special problem of legitimacy facing health plans that make limit setting decisions any more than there is a problem of legitimacy facing automobile manufacturers when they make decisions regarding product features and design. If a car manufacturer makes cost-cutting decisions that affect the quality of a product, the market provides a mechanism for putting a price on that decision and allowing consumers to match their preferences with the price of products. Although some safety features of automobiles are mandated by law, and consumer protection legislation provides some further defense against duplicitous practices by car manufacturers, we already have similar protections in the case of health care through insurance law and tort litigation. Beyond that, the market—for cars or health insurance—provides an efficient mechanism for matching consumer preferences to market share. Accordingly, if consumers do not like the limit-setting decisions of a medical insurer, they are free to purchase other medical insurance that better meets their preferences. The obligation of the insurer, like the auto manufacturer, is to be honest and forthright about the features of the product, eschewing deception. There is no further obligation to provide access to a process of decision-making to make sure it meets some standard of fairness that really plays no role in a market economy.

The car purchase analogy aims to show that consumer choices in a market for medical insurance confer legitimacy since they involve consent. The analogy fails for several reasons, some having to do with special features of the medical marketplace, others with features of the U.S. health care system, and still others from having their foundations deep in considerations of distributive justice.

Uncertainty is a much greater factor in markets for medical insurance than it is in markets for autos (Arrow, 1963). With cars, we have a good idea just what our needs are: we know how many passengers we will have to carry, what kinds of commuting or cargo carrying we will do, and what our style of driving is. We also have reasonably good information about outcomes: *Consumer Reports* or its equivalent tells us which cars get what kinds of mileage under what conditions, which have better safety records, which have better service records (with detailed ratings for different aspects of the car), and which have higher customer satisfaction and resale value. We have much greater trouble anticipating our needs for health care if we have no obvious history of problems, and if we do have such a history, we may be excluded from purchasing insurance, that is, from shopping around, because of medical underwriting practices of insurers. We also have not yet developed an adequate technology for reporting on the quality of health plans through good measures of outcomes, though new measurement techniques are being developed.

Features of the design of our health care system also undercut the car purchase analogy. Most Americans receive their health insurance through decisions made by their employers, who select the health plans to which employees are attached. We do not buy our private cars through fleet purchases made by our employers. The piece of market ideology that says that people consent with their purchases to the limits that insurers impose on them has no grip on the actual situation of most insured Americans, who cannot practically "vote with their dollars" even if, in theory, that would constitute consent. If they are lucky enough to have insurance at all, it comes with the job, and the only choice they have is to change jobs, if they can. Nor should we say that we consent to the terms of the medical insurance policy because we consent to having our employer select our insurance coverage for us. Although some employers may seek a plan that produces good value for money, it would be naive to think that an employer's interest in containing costs always can be translated without controversy into an employee's interest in accepting compromises in coverage. The employer is not the employee's fiduciary agent.

In part as a result of the backlash against managed care in the 1990s, a trend has emerged to give more choice to employees. Instead of choosing among whatever health plans are offered by their employers, employees would be given a sum of money (a "defined contribution") earmarked for health insurance. Employees who chose an option that cost more than the defined contribution would be responsible for the incremental cost. Under some forms of this scheme, employees who chose an option that cost less could keep the money or put it to another use.

Although under this system employees would not be constrained by the health plan options provided by their employers, they would be constrained by their ability to pay for options that cost more than the defined contribution. Higher paid employees will be able to afford a richer package of benefits. There is a significant risk that the basic benefit that can be purchased with the defined contribution will diminish in quality. Our claim is that the limits set by these cost differences must themselves be justifiable by rationales fair minded people can accept, and this requires transparency that goes beyond what market choice provides. Without accountability for reasonableness the new trend offers the semblance of legitimacy through choice, not the real thing.

The car purchase analogy fails for a deeper, moral reason as well: As we claimed in the previous chapter, we have a widely recognized obligation to meet people's medical needs, within reasonable resource constraints, but we do not have a social obligation to meet people's preferences or needs for autos.

Nevertheless, there is something useful in the idea of market accountability, namely, its requirement that people be adequately informed about the choices they do face—or the limited options they have. The fair process we describe in the next chapter builds on this goal of adequate information and carries it an important step further. It will turn out that it is crucial to understand the rationales for limit-setting decisions and not simply the options that limits give us.

THE APPEAL TO DISTRIBUTIVE PRINCIPLES

The central idea behind this alternative is the belief that, with proper philosophical inquiry, we will achieve consensus on principles of justice, or more specific distributive principles, that will tell us which limits are fair. With such clear principles, we would not need to rely on fair process to resolve disputes or establish legitimacy. It may seem ornery of us to devote the previous chapter to showing that principles of justice oblige us to meet health care needs fairly and then to turn around in this chapter and argue that the principles we have just defended fail to answer key questions about fair distribution. Ornery or not, that is what we believe. We must rely on fair process because acceptable general principles of justice fail to give us determinate answers about fair allocation and because we have no consensus on more fine-grained principles that do. Of course, in due time, philosophical inquiry may lead us to the desired principles. It will, in any case, improve our deliberation within a fair process, but it cannot obviate the need for such a process.

Unsolved Rationing Problems

We begin by returning to a problem we briefly mentioned in Chapter 1: How much priority should we give to treating the sickest or most disabled patients?

To start with, imagine two extreme positions. At one extreme is the view that we should give complete priority to treating the worst-off patients. One might think that the fair-equality-of-opportunity principle, or other views that give priority to those with the worst opportunity, would lead us to this extreme position. At the other extreme is a view that says we should give priority to whatever treatment produces the greatest net health benefit (or greatest net health benefit per dollar spent) regardless of which patients we treat. Some utilitarian views are committed to this principle, and it is embedded in standard methods for calculating the cost-effectiveness of alternative treatments.

These extreme positions would have different implications for specific resource allocation decisions. Suppose that a health plan or a public agency operated under a fixed budget and could invest a million dollars in providing treatment A to one type of patient or treatment B to another group of patients, and suppose that the investment in equipment and personnel required that we devote the million dollars to either A or B and not to some of each. The extreme view that says we give complete priority to the worst off settles the matter by determining whether patients needing A are worse off than patients needing B. No attention is then paid to what the outcomes are for either group of patients. The other extreme view settles the matter by asking only what the outcomes are: we should invest in whichever technology produces the net maximum benefit, regardless of how badly off people are before they are treated.

In practice, most people reject both extreme positions. This fact emerges in both moral and empirical examination of these kinds of cases (Nord, 1999). Though many people end up agreeing that there should be *some,* but not complete, priority given to those who are sickest, there is also considerable disagreement. A distinct, but small, minority adheres to one or the other extreme position. Those in the middle differ in their degree of commitment to helping those who are worst off. They may want to help the worst off, provided the benefits others must then sacrifice are not too great, but there is a range of beliefs about what level of sacrifice is too great.

Disputants about these hypothetical cases are quite willing to back their conclusions with reasons. Some will say, for example, "Although patients needing B are being asked to forgo a significant benefit, I simply cannot turn my back on patients needing A, since they are so badly off." In response, someone else will say, "I hate to abandon patients needing A, but I simply cannot expect patients needing B to sacrifice a much greater benefit just because those needing A start off so poorly."

Once we abandon either extreme position, we are in an area where general principles give no guidance. Therefore, we need a fair process to resolve disputes among all the various views.

Similar points emerge if we consider this distinct problem: When should we allow an aggregation of modest benefits to larger numbers of people to outweigh more significant benefits to fewer people (Daniels, 1993; Kamm, 1987, 1993)? For example, when, if ever, should curing a great number of minor headaches outweigh adding 30 healthy years to a small number of lives?

One extreme position is the view that we should maximize aggregate health benefits, allowing all possible ways of aggregating them. The utilitarian underpinnings of standard cost-effectiveness analysis may drive us to this extreme. An opposite extreme is that we should never allow the aggregation of benefits, even when we are considering benefits of the same type; we should not, for example, save five lives in preference to saving three, except by lottery.

In the United States, we have an actual example of the public rejection of the extreme view that any aggregation is permissible in the pursuit of maximum benefits. In June 1990, the Oregon Health Services Commission released a list of treatment/condition pairs ranked by a cost/benefit calculation. Critics were quick to seize on rankings that seemed completely counterintuitive. (Other critics argue the problem arose because the commission used crude numbers.) In the commission's ranking, capping teeth was ranked higher, that is, more important than, appendectomy (Hadorn, 1991). The reason was simple: an appendectomy then cost about $4000, many times the cost of capping a tooth. Simply aggregating the net medical benefit of many capped teeth yielded a net benefit greater than that produced by one appendectomy. Ultimately, the commission revised its methodology, placing whole categories of services that delivered major benefits to seriously ill patients out of reach of this form of universal aggregating.

The aggregation problem is a case in which the equal opportunity account, like the broader family of views we noted earlier, ends up giving answers that are indeterminate. Our account focuses on using resources to promote normal functioning as a specific, limited way of protecting the opportunity range of individuals. It will have to pay attention to the significant gains in opportunity that come from concentrating resources on those with significant deficits, and it may plausibly refuse to allow those gains to be outweighed by many trivial gains to others. It must also not ignore the loss of opportunity for those with moderate conditions, and therefore it must permit some kinds of aggregation. Unfortunately, it remains too indeterminate to be of help in resolving disputes about which aggregations are compatible with the objective of best protecting fair equality of opportunity under resource constraints.

One further type of problem illustrates the same point again: How much should we favor producing the *best outcome* with our limited resources as opposed to giving people a *fair chance* at deriving some benefit from them? A utilitarian account might opt directly for maximizing expected payoff, directing resources toward the patient group with the greatest expected benefit. A more egalitarian approach, or one that gave more weight to the subjective value that each person would place on whatever level of benefit might be possible for her, might favor a lottery giving equal chances to all who might in any way benefit.

In the philosophical literature on this topic, a number of middle positions have been defended, including calls for proportional or weighted lotteries. In such a lottery, people with greater expected benefits are given more chances to get the desired treatment than those with lesser expected benefits (Brock, 1988, Kamm, 1993). There is an element of arbitrariness to the precision that results from such weighted lotteries since we have no guidance from any plausible theory telling us just how much weight to give to providing equal or fair chances versus favoring outcomes. (This arbitrariness would be removed or seem less troublesome if the weightings given in the lottery were themselves the results of a fair, deliberative process.)

Further Moral Inquiry

Perhaps we are looking in the wrong place when we look to general accounts of distributive justice for principles that would allow us to resolve these three unsolved rationing problems. If we need more fine-grained principles to apply to cases like these, perhaps we should start with the cases and work our way toward finding acceptable principles for them. We need a different kind of moral methodology and should not throw up our hands because quite general principles fail us.

The most systematic and ingenious philosophical effort to work from cases to appropriate principles is found in Frances Kamm's (1993) work. Rather than examine real-world resource allocation problems, with all their complexity, she proposes we examine carefully selected hypothetical cases that sound quite fantastical to nonphilosophers. For example, we are asked to imagine a runaway trolley that will strike and kill or injure X number of people if it is not redirected onto another track, where it will kill or injure Y number of people. By varying these simplified cases, which function as thought experiments, she hopes to uncover the underlying moral structure or "inner program," as she puts it, of our beliefs. Her results yield somewhat more fine-grained reasons and principles about aggregation than the kind of extreme views we noted. We definitely view some utilities or benefits we might gain as trivial and incomparable to those involved in saving lives. We would not, for example, decide which of two people to save because, by saving one rather than the other, we can additionally cure a sore throat. Losing a leg or arm, however, is a significant loss, and her examination of hypothetical cases yields the judgment that we rightly give higher proportional chances to saving a life and a leg than to just saving a life. Even though we would prefer to save a single life to a single leg, she concludes that we should agree to give some proportional chance to saving many legs rather than one life. At the macro level of resource allocation, Kamm continues, we should be willing to forego helping a few people who might die if we did not cure their diseases in order to, instead, help a much larger number of people who would lose legs.

Philosophical inquiry of the sort Kamm uses—or other approaches, based on real, not hypothetical, examples—promises to yield middle-level reasons and principles that can guide us to fair allocations of resources. One risk of her approach is that she may base her principles on idiosyncratic judgments about cases. Other people may not make the same judgment, or may not be able to make any confident judgment at all about such hypothetical cases. To agree with her conclusions is to agree to many assumptions underlying her method that other philosophers do not accept (Daniels, 1998b). Nevertheless, one benefit of her approach is that it forces careful deliberation about reasons and how we justify them, and it suggests that some progress on publicly justifiable principles is at least possible, with adequate philosophical investigation.

We make a modest claim. Whether fine-grained principles such as those Kamm argues for could ultimately provide the basis for a consensus on fair distribution, they are not likely to provide that consensus in the short- or mid-term. Given that we have no prior consensus on adequate principles for these rationing problems, moreover, they cannot substitute for a fair process for resolving disputes. This kind of inquiry, however, provides an excellent input into a fair, deliberative process. Encouraging this kind of investigation and the dissemination of its results can only enhance the quality of deliberation about limits in whatever fair process is constructed.

"MAJORITY RULE" AND FAIR PROCESS

Society cannot dispel the fairness and legitimacy problems by claiming that buyers choose the limits acceptable to them in an insurance market. Neither can it settle disputes by appealing to a consensus on appropriate distributive principles— we lack such a consensus. We simply cannot achieve legitimacy and fairness without a fair process. But if we must rely on fair process, what is the mystery? Citizens use democratic procedures and majority rule, directly or indirectly, to resolve other policy disputes. Why not the same solution to limit setting for health care?

We agree that a democratic process should be the ultimate authority for settling disputes about limit setting in health care, but we also believe that we must understand that process in a particular way if it is to have legitimacy as a way of resolving moral disputes about the distribution of health care. Some of the conditions we describe in the next chapter as necessary elements of fair process draw heavily on a particular conception of democratic legitimacy. This conception emphasizes the deliberative component of democratic process, not merely a procedural appeal to majority rule. In order to set the groundwork for the conditions we argue for in the next chapter, we here briefly describe the underlying philosophical debate about the legitimacy of democratic processes (Cohen, 1996a, 1996b, 1994; Rawls, 1993; Sunstein, 1993; Gutmann & Thompson, 1996; Estlund, 1997).

What gives majority (or plurality) rule its legitimacy as a procedure for resolving moral disputes about public policy and the design of institutions? One prominent answer, sometimes referred to as the "aggregative" conception of democracy (Cohen, 1996a, p. 14) holds that the procedure is fair and acquires legitimacy simply because it counts everyone's interests equally in the voting process; each counts for one, not more or less. Adult persons are presumed to be the best judges of their own interests and can present and advance them in the political process.

Something important seems to be left out of this proceduralist view of the virtues of aggregation through voting. It allows us to compel people to abide by a majority rule, even where there are matters of fundamental moral disagreement, simply by aggregating the preferences of the voters, whatever they happen to be.[1] If we had a large group and the option of buying only one flavor of ice cream, vanilla or chocolate, we might settle the dispute by voting. We might think that aggregating preferences through the mechanism of voting was a way to achieve the greatest net satisfaction of preferences. If most people prefer chocolate, then we get the greatest aggregate satisfaction of preferences by buying chocolate. Everyone's interests are counted, including those who prefer vanilla, since the frustration of the vanilla lovers is offset by the greater pleasure of the chocolate lovers.

Abiding by a majority decision that compels people to act in ways that counter their fundamental beliefs about what is morally right is not simply like frustrating a taste for vanilla ice cream, however. Even a craving for vanilla is not to be assimilated to a moral conviction. Settling moral disputes simply by aggregating preferences seems to ignore some fundamental differences between the nature of values and commitments to them and tastes or preferences.

The aggregative conception seems insensitive to how we ideally would like to resolve moral disputes, namely through argument and deliberation. We expect people to offer reasons and arguments for their moral views, and we hope that the better arguments will prove persuasive. We want to be shown what is right by an appeal to reasons that we consider convincing. If a good moral argument persuades us that our original belief about what is right is in fact incorrect, we may be chagrined, but we are (or should be) grateful as well. We have been spared doing what is wrong. It is more important to end up knowing what is right and doing it, given our motivation to act in ways that we can justify morally, than it is to get our way.

This observation helps to explain why we are not satisfied in cases of moral disagreement simply to be told, "a majority of people think otherwise." The problem is not simply that the majority will keep us from getting our way (as it would be if we preferred vanilla), but that majorities can be morally wrong and may make us do the wrong thing. In addition, they may be moved by reasons that minorities cannot even accept as relevant to resolving the dispute.

The aggregative account fails as an account of the legitimacy of a democratic procedure because it ignores the way reasons play a role in our deliberations about what is right. An alternative account of how a procedure such as majority rule acquires legitimacy depends on emphasizing the deliberative process that may conclude in a vote. Specifically, it imposes some constraints on the kinds of reasons that can play a role in that deliberation. Not just any reasons will do.

Reasons must reflect the fact that all parties to a decision are viewed as seeking terms of fair cooperation that all can accept as reasonable. Where their well-being or fundamental liberties or other matters of fundamental value are involved and at risk, people should not be expected to accept binding terms of cooperation that rest on reasons they cannot view as acceptable types of reasons. For example, reasons that rest on matters of religious faith will not meet this condition. Reasonable people differ in their religious, philosophical, and moral views, and yet we must seek terms of fair cooperation that rest on justifications acceptable to all.

Suppose that a deliberation appeals only to reasons that all can recognize as acceptable or relevant, but that consensus about an outcome is still not achieved. To settle the practical matter, we rely on a majority vote. What can be said in favor of reliance on this voting procedure that could not be said on the purely proceduralist view—a vote not preceded by a comparable deliberation?

Relying on a majority vote to settle the matter has one advantage over the purely proceduralist (or aggregative) account: the minority is not being compelled to do something for reasons it thinks irrelevant or inappropriate—even if it does not accept the weight or balance given to various considerations by the majority. In the aggregative view, the minority has to accept the fact that it loses only because more people prefer an alternative, for whatever reasons. In the deliberative democracy view, the minority can at least assure itself that the preference of the majority rests on the kind of reason that even the minority must acknowledge appropriately plays a role in the deliberation. The majority does not exercise brute power of preference but is constrained by having to seek reasons for its view that are justifiable to all who seek mutually justifiable terms of cooperation.

The constraints on reasons involved in the account of fair process we offer in Chapter 4 have a similar effect. This is true even though the decision-making procedure is itself often not a democratic one, especially when it takes place in a privately controlled health plan. Still, if the private health plan reveals, through a pattern of public reason-giving, that its decisions rest on the kinds of reasons all can consider relevant to deciding how to meet varied patient needs under reasonable resource constraints, then even those who disagree with the plan's specific decisions should acknowledge they are reasonable and arguably aimed at producing fair outcomes. If all affected by these decisions acknowledge that much, then decision makers would be well on their way toward earning or achieving legitimacy for their process. We are getting ahead of our story, however, and should return to consider one further alternative.

EMPIRICAL ETHICS AND A COST-VALUE METHODOLOGY

The fourth alternative to constructing a fair process is to develop an ethically sensitive, empirically based methodology for making resource allocation decisions. If the methodology incorporated social values, as measured by social scientists, then decision makers using it could be confident that the results would reflect what the public considers acceptable. Such a methodology would be usable at many levels in a system and would yield results that are publicly accountable.

Traditional cost-effectiveness (or "cost-utility") analysis was intended to be an empirically based methodology that was transparent in its reliance on evidence. The technique requires converting all effects on both mortality and morbidity into one outcome measure (such as the Quality Adjusted Life Year [QALY] or the Disability Adjusted Life Year [DALY]). Then all costs are calculated and a ratio of costs-to-effects can be calculated. With proper standardization, the ratios can then be used to compare a broad range of interventions on quite different categories of patients.

Unfortunately, that methodology carries with it some morally controversial—and many insist, unacceptable—assumptions (Brock, 1998; Nord, 1999). One key assumption with troubling consequences is that a unit of benefit, such as a QALY or DALY, is worth just as much, regardless of who gets it. Yet, it may well matter morally to us that someone who is much more seriously ill gets the extra benefit rather than someone less ill, or we may not be willing to aggregate minor benefits across large populations and outweigh, in the aggregate, major benefits, such as saving lives, for a few. As we noted earlier, cost-effectiveness rankings of medical treatments led to publicly unacceptable results in Oregon's attempt to establish funding priorities for Medicaid.

It might be possible, however, to modify a cost-effectiveness analysis so that it could avoid this kind of moral objection. We might, through empirical study, provide "ethical weightings" for outcomes so that they reflected public values about the kinds of trade-offs involved in medical resource allocation (Menzel, Gold, Nord et al., 1999). Alternatively, we might abandon traditional cost-effectiveness methodology and substitute for it an empirically based "cost-value" approach (Nord, 1999).

How might we measure people's values so that we can tell what kinds of trade-offs they would approve in resource allocation decisions? One proposal is to survey people by asking them about the "person trade-offs" they are willing to make when they face hypothetical forced choices as medical resource allocators (Nord, 1999). (This approach is a variation on a standard economic approach seeking "indifference" points, or curves, reflecting when an individual finds two benefits or outcomes equivalent.) Suppose we know that we can only do A or B; that is, we can fund one kind of medical service or another. (Often, however, we can do some of each.) Treatment A affects people with a more serious prior condition than the people treated by B. We can ask people when they would trade treating X number of people by A for treating Y number of people by B. The claim is that these person–trade-off questions uncover directly the value to people of one service over another, given the information people have about initial health states and health outcomes. With improvements in the survey methods, we could gather information about a broad range of trade-offs people are willing to make.

There are important concerns about this methodology and the values we can extract from it. Its proponents are aware, for example, that the values people assign are very much affected by the way questions are framed, giving rise to "starting point biases." If the same surveys are repeated, there is variation in the answers, meaning "test-retest validity" is problematic. There is also considerable variation in the responses people give within a population, and there is evidence these variations correlate with attitudes, for example, with political affiliation.[2] Ignoring this variation by using a median within the range of answers people give risks ignoring the moral disagreement underlying it. This problem raises a serious worry about the degree to which the empirical results could be used to substitute for actual deliberation by decision makers.

Suppose, however, that we find considerable convergence in a population (or subgroup) on the magnitudes involved in trade-offs. What should we make of it? Should we view it as a prevalent taste or preference, the equivalent of a predominant taste for chocolate over vanilla ice cream? Or are the responses the result of a deliberative or reflective process in which people weigh various reasons, principles, and intuitions about particular cases and arrive at a coherent set of moral beliefs that for them is justified?

We risk having uncovered only tastes, not values, if we carry out a straightforward survey of attitudes toward trade-offs. We may be getting at reasons and values if we instead develop and deploy more complex methods. For example, we might lead subjects in these surveys through a series of questions that import arguments and reasons that might be the basis for making these trades. This complex technique, which is quite demanding, begins to approximate the sort of philosophical exploration involved when students are led through the complexities of these issues by posing various hypothetical cases (cf. Nord, 1999; cf. Kamm, 1993). Such an approach is more likely to uncover some evidence about what *reasons* people give weight to, and not simply their unconsidered *tastes*.

One quite general challenge to this empirical approach to characterizing the public's values is the following "anthropological objection." For the sake of argument, let us set aside the methodological worries we have been discussing. Then we can still ask, "*So what* if we happen to have these preferences that empirical researchers call values? *Should* we hold them? We could, after all, have had others. No doubt other cultures, or subgroups within our own, will have different preferences. Can we defend them morally, or can we only say, this is what *we* happen to prefer?" The objection invites us to place the information the empirical investigation gives us in a more deliberative context, which is exactly what we are proposing.

There is another way to think about the results of this kind of empirical investigation using the person–trade-off approach. Leaving aside methodological worries about reliability and validity, could we view them as a substitute or proxy for democratic voting on these matters? Obviously, we cannot put all resource allocation decisions to direct democratic referenda; nor should we. But, if we had good evidence about what the public believed about these matters, then we might be able to construct a socially acceptable table, giving weights to types of outcomes, and then use this table as a proxy for more direct democratic decision-making. Policy makers responsible for resource allocation decisions could try to establish legitimacy for their decisions by saying that they reflect what the public is known to believe should be done.

This proxy-democratic defense of the person–trade-off approach must be rejected if is taken literally. Simple democratic voting itself, or the proxy for voting embodied in the person–trade-off method, itself faces the objections that we earlier raised, at least when we are concerned with moral disagreements. Merely aggregating preferences through voting or surveying ends up making majority might determine what is right, with no real constraints on the kinds of reasons that play a role in the decision. In moral disagreements, we want people to bring reasons to bear in an effort to persuade each other. We want a deliberative process that takes seriously the considerations people bring into a dispute. A dispute resolved by democratic procedures after careful deliberation about the various reasons put forward on both sides has in its favor the fact that even losers will know that their beliefs about what is right were taken seriously by others. This deliberative component of fair democratic process is missing if we simply think of the weightings generated by person–trade-offs as a proxy for voting.

Nevertheless, if people responsible for decision-making at various levels within a health-care system view the results of a refined person–trade-off study as an input to their deliberation, then we can retain the deliberative component of fair democratic process. This is the more plausible scenario for using this information.[3] We believe that including the results of unmodified cost-effectiveness analyses in a deliberative process could also be of some use. In a fully deliberative context, the disturbing—and many would say unfair—implications of cost-effectiveness analysis could at least be introduced and the value of the analysis assessed in light of those concerns. In the absence of an open deliberative process, however, cost-effectiveness analysis carries with it the risk that important distributive concerns will be ignored. Without corrective deliberation, cost-effectiveness analysis is an inadequate framework for decision making.

CRITICS OF PUBLICITY

To finish providing the groundwork for our approach, and to reply even more directly to the Implicit Rationer, we need to respond to a more general line of criticism of public accountability based on the view that explicit limit setting is impractical and too socially divisive. Open, public, limit-setting decisions have costs. They involve openly favoring some claims against others, possibly in life-or-death situations. We can expect losers—whoever they turn out to be—to fight these decisions, and when limits cause suffering to identifiable individuals and groups, the public may also protest against them. The costs of publicity may include threatening important public values. In a celebrated book, Calabresi and Bobbit (1978) argue that the costs may include eroding such values as the sanctity of life and that somewhat more indirect methods of decision-making might accomplish the same distribution but without the public costs. These considerations lead the Implicit Rationer to conclude that public decision-making would be infeasible.

The Implicit Rationer is making a two-part argument that combines sociological description and ethical analysis. At the level of description, the Implicit Rationer cites the practical burdens and social conflict explicit rationing may cause. At the level of ethical analysis, the Implicit Rationer argues that when we weigh all costs and benefits, nonpublic rationing methods are sometimes morally superior to public ones (Klein, 1995; Mechanic, 1997a; but cf. Mechanic, 2000).

These objections deserve a more extensive reply than can be given here, and we shall return to this issue in later chapters, but enough has been said to offer an overview of our response. To the charge that publicity is infeasible, we reply that nonpublicity is also infeasible for a very basic reason: it does not work. The public is too suspicious, especially of for-profit private organizations, but even of bureaucrats in publicly administered systems, to accept implicit limit setting. As shown by the massive anti-managed-care backlash in the United States, all decisions are viewed with skepticism, and many are opposed through litigation or even legislation. Whereas nonpublicity has been tried and has failed, however, publicity has not yet been seriously attempted.

To the claim that nonpublicity is preferable to publicity because it better preserves important public values, we reply that nonpublicity risks undercutting the public sense that fairness obtains in the system. A public increasingly accustomed to using the Internet to bypass experts and seek out its own information is not willing to accept decisions on the basis of authority. In this climate, publicity may be a necessary condition for public acceptance of limit setting, provided it is done fairly and legitimately. Again, whereas nonpublicity has failed as a solution to the fairness and legitimacy problems, little effort has been made to see what effects publicity produces.

What would it mean to say that publicity "worked" whereas nonpublicity for limit-setting decisions "failed"? We can recast this as the following question:

Under what conditions should the public begin to view health plans and public agencies as a legitimate locus for making limit-setting decisions? We answer this question in the next chapter and illustrate early lessons gained from applying our answer in Chapters 5–9.

NOTES

1. Cohen notes that an aggregative view might arguably be extended to give some protection against outcomes that involved discrimination against those who are targets of stereotyping or hostility, e.g., against people with disabilities or racial minorities. A process that allowed simple aggregation of those preferences arguably does not give people equal consideration and so violates its own rationale (Cohen, 1996b, p.15).

2. Nord presents evidence for differences that vary with Norwegian political party affiliations in the following table:

Percentage of utilitarian preferences in five different choice contexts

CONTEXT	I	II	III	IV	V
Conservatives	52	21	50	20	27
Social Democrats	18	11	28	8	15

(Nord, 1999, p. 130, Table 16)

To control for framing effects, Nord suggests subjects be taken through various steps in which they are exposed to different arguments that might be relevant to the exercise, but he notes that identifying the ethical positions the subjects want to adopt influences the answers they give.

3. Eric Nord (personal communication) has suggested that this is how he believes this kind of information should in fact be used—as an input to a fair, deliberative process.

4

ACCOUNTABILITY FOR REASONABLENESS

There is no escaping the need to construct a fair process for setting limits to health care. Other ways of addressing or avoiding the legitimacy and fairness problems— market accountability, the philosopher's alternative, the majority rule approach, or the survey of public attitudes—give us important clues to the components of such a process, but do not substitute for it. We must now try to characterize the key features of fair process in more detail. In this chapter, we describe the conditions that must be met in order for both private organizations, such as health plans, and public agencies to be accepted as legitimate moral authorities for distributing health care fairly.

After considering some objections to the moral and other costs of publicity, we argued in the previous chapter that public accountability must be a central feature of such a process. In fact, in the backlash against managed care in the United States in the late 1990s, public accountability became the battle cry of health care reform. It was proclaimed in President Clinton's Consumer's Bill of Rights, in the Principles for Consumer Protection proposed by a coalition of managed care organizations and consumers,[1] in many legislative proposals introduced at the state level, and in accreditation standards by the National Committee on Quality Assurance. In all these contexts, public accountability meant robust disclosure of relevant information about health plan benefits and performance, as well as a demand for due process in the form of grievance and appeals procedures, sometimes combined with a right to sue the health plan.

Public accountability has obvious appeal. Disclosure informs our consent, not only as to treatments but to our choice of providers and plans. Informed choice expresses our autonomy and is the lever that pushes markets to work responsively and efficiently.

There are, however, two distinct notions of public accountability: market accountability and accountability for reasonableness. It is important to distinguish them because they are central to quite different views about what constitutes a fair and just health care system. In our mixed public and private system, both kinds of accountability are necessary.

Market accountability is the idea that information about performance and options must be made available to purchasers and enrollees in health plans so that they can effectively make choices among plans, clinicians, and treatments. Only with such information can consumers and purchasers leverage providers to improve quality of care and be responsive to patient needs and desires. Nevertheless, as we argued in the previous chapter, market accountability alone cannot solve the legitimacy and fairness problems. In the United States, only half of all insured workers have any choice of health plan. Further, once people are ill and actually become better informed about their needs, they no longer have mobility among plans. The market also offers no assurance that available plans constitute a fair and reasonable array of choices.

Accountability for reasonableness is the idea that the reasons or rationales for important limit-setting decisions should be publicly available. In addition, these reasons must be ones that "fair-minded" people can agree are relevant to pursuing appropriate patient care under necessary resource constraints (Daniels & Sabin, 1998b). This is our central thesis, and it needs some explanation.

By "fair-minded," we do not simply mean our friends or people who just happen to agree with us. We mean people who in principle seek to cooperate with others on terms they can justify to each other. Indeed, fair-minded people accept rules of the game—or sometimes seek rule changes—that promote the game's essential skills and the excitement their use produces. For example, they want rules that permit blocking in football, but not clipping or grabbing facemasks, because they want to encourage teamwork and skill and not the mere advantage that comes from imposing injuries. Of course, having rules of a game that fair-minded people accept does not eliminate all controversy about their application. It does, however, narrow the scope of controversy and the methods for adjudicating them.

In the "game" of delivering health care, whether in public or private insurance schemes, fair-minded people will seek reasons ("rules") they can accept as relevant to meeting consumers' or citizens' needs fairly under resource constraints. As in football, the rules shape a conception of the common good that is the goal of cooperation within plans, even when plans compete. In health care delivery, as in football, some will seek mere advantage by ignoring the rules, or by seeking rules that advantage only them, and there will be disagreement about how to apply the rules. Still, the fair-minded search for mutually acceptable rules narrows the scope of disagreement and provides the grounds on which disputes can be adjudicated.

Accountability for reasonableness obviously goes beyond what is required by market accountability alone. Market accountability requires only that we be informed about the options insurers give us and about their record of performance. Accountability for reasonableness requires that we also have access to the reasons for the insurer's (or government agency's) policies and decisions, and that these policies and decisions be based on the kinds of reasons fair-minded people consider relevant to the challenge of providing high quality care to all within limited resources. Market accountability leaves it to the consumer to infer from the choices available what commitments a health plan has to responsible patient-centered care. Accountability for reasonableness requires that there be a way to revisit decisions when their application in specific cases is problematic and a mechanism to revise and improve decisions over time as we learn from experience. In these ways, accountability for reasonableness requires the health plan or public agency to be explicit about its value commitments and allows all of us to learn what those commitments imply and to challenge them in a thoughtful way.

FOUR CONDITIONS

The following four conditions make more precise the notion of accountability for reasonableness (Daniels & Sabin, 1997):

1. **Publicity Condition:** Decisions regarding both direct and indirect limits to care and their rationales must be publicly accessible.
2. **Relevance Condition:** The rationales for limit-setting decisions should aim to provide a *reasonable* explanation of how the organization seeks to provide "value for money" in meeting the varied health needs of a defined population under reasonable resource constraints. Specifically, a rationale will be reasonable if it appeals to evidence, reasons, and principles that are accepted as relevant by fair-minded people who are disposed to finding mutually justifiable terms of cooperation.
3. **Revision and Appeals Condition:** There must be mechanisms for challenge and dispute resolution regarding limit-setting decisions, and, more broadly, opportunities for revision and improvement of policies in the light of new evidence or arguments.
4. **Regulative Condition:** There is either voluntary or public regulation of the process to ensure that conditions 1–3 are met.

These four conditions capture the central necessary elements of a solution to the legitimacy and fairness problems. The Publicity Condition requires openness or publicity; that is, transparency with regard to the reasons for a decision. The Relevance Condition sets constraints on the kinds of reasons that can play a role in the rationale; it recognizes the fundamental interest in finding a justification all can accept as reasonable. The Revision Condition makes learning from experience and responding to disagreements a central component of decision-making. The Regulative Condition puts teeth into the others. Taken together, the four conditions bring managed care decision-making out of a mysterious black box and make it possible to assess health plan and public agency decisions in the light of wider societal views about what fairness requires They connect health-plan decisions to a broader educative and deliberative democratic process.[2]

For private health plans and public agencies to acquire and sustain legitimacy for their limit-setting decisions, they must see themselves, and be seen by others, as contributors to a broader deliberative process that they constructively embrace. The four conditions contribute to a solution to the legitimacy and fairness problems by placing private health plans—arguably a harder case than public agencies—visibly in that role. Embracing these conditions and the way in which they connect internal decisions to broader, public deliberation clearly carries many of these organizations beyond the dominant perceptions they currently have of their organizational and (in many cases) corporate culture, for it makes them accountable to more than their own boards of directors and—if they have them—stockholders. In an intensely competitive environment, embracing these conditions may be easier for associations of organizations than for individual health plans, though it may also be possible to show there is some market value in having a visible record of commitment to patient-oriented decision-making.[3]

THE PUBLICITY CONDITION: PUBLIC RATIONALES

The Publicity Condition requires that rationales for decisions such as coverage for new technologies or the contents of a drug formulary be publicly accessible to clinicians, patients, and would-be subscribers—or citizens in a publicly administered system. To see what this condition means in practice, consider how one leading health plan in 1993 disseminated its coverage decision for biosynthetic growth hormone. In a medical director's letter distributed to all clinicians, the policy stated that growth hormone treatment would be covered (for those with a contractual drug benefit) only for children with growth hormone deficiency or Turner's syndrome. No explanation was offered for the restrictions in coverage to these categories of patients. We compared this coverage statement to those made by several other health plans; they placed similar coverage restrictions on growth hormone treatment and also failed to say why.[4]

Why insist that the rationale for limitations on coverage, and not simply the decisions themselves, be made public, for example, in an instrument such as a medical director's letter? The point of offering the rationale is made clearer when we imagine the parents of a child projected to have very short stature who want the treatment, but whose child does not fit the patient selection criteria. What can be said to them that would make the limitation seem reasonable and based on considerations that take the welfare of patients into account?

When the committee of the health plan charged with making a coverage decision for growth hormone originally made its decision, it deliberated quite carefully about two reasons for the restrictions, drawing on literature reviews and expert opinions. First, growth hormone therapy had not been shown to be effective in increasing ultimate adult height in short children who were not deficient in growth hormone. Second, independently of the question of effectiveness, the committee considered that, while extreme short stature may be disadvantageous, in the absence of growth hormone deficiency, it should not be considered an illness and therefore would not be eligible for treatment in the insurance benefit package.

A failure to be clear about these reasons in either coverage committee minutes or the disseminated coverage decision has important consequences. The first reason has obvious relevance that anxious parents must take into account, but if the treatment's efficacy were later demonstrated, and the second reason had not been publicly stated and explicitly defended, it might seem that coverage would have to be provided. The distinction between treatments for disease or disability and therapies that enhance otherwise normal traits is crucial in other coverage decisions, and so, when used, it ought to be stated clearly and explicitly defended. For example, it is central in decisions about coverage for donor oocyte in vitro fertilization ("donor egg") for postmenopausal women and in restrictions on breast reduction surgery. Consequently, being explicit about the underlying reasoning is a chance to demonstrate the coherence and consistency of an overall policy toward coverage. It is a chance to demonstrate that there is a commitment to an even-handed appeal to reasons and principles, so that relevant similarities and differences in particular cases are recognized and attended to.

Analogy to Case Law

One important effect of making the reasons for coverage decisions public is that, over time, the pattern of such decisions will resemble a type of case law. The virtues of a case-law model will help us see that the benefits of the Publicity Condition are both internal to health plans committed to it, leading to more efficient, coherent, and fairer decisions over time, and external, since the emerging "case law" can strengthen broader public deliberation and contribute to the perceived legitimacy of decision makers.

One important requirement of fairness is that similar cases be dealt with similarly and that differential treatment be justified by relevant reasons. A body of case law establishes the presumption that, if some individuals have been treated one way because they fall under a reasonable interpretation of the relevant policies or rationales, similar individuals should be treated the same way in subsequent cases. The earlier decision reflects a *commitment* to continue to act on the cited reasons and rationales in future similar cases. There is a presumption that the earlier, reason-based deliberation about a case will be applied to similar cases in the present.

There are two ways to rebut this presumption that a subsequent case should be treated similarly to an earlier one. The least disruptive rebuttal involves showing that the new case differs in relevant and important ways from the earlier one, justifying different treatment. A much more disruptive rebuttal would involve rejecting the reasons or principles embodied in the earlier case. Sometimes, such a revision of past policy is justifiable and required. The respect for past commitments embodied in case law does not mean that past errors of judgments cannot be corrected by new deliberation. Case law does not imply past infallibility, but it does imply giving careful consideration to why earlier decision makers made the choices they did. Since treating a new case differently from a (similar) old one thus involves acknowledging a change and perhaps an earlier error in policy, the case law model demands a clear rationale and new avowal of principles and commitments in order to avoid the appearance of inconsistency or deliberate unfairness in treatment.

Case law thus involves a form of institutional reflective equilibrium—movement between deliberation and practice, checking one against the other (Rawls, 1971; Daniels, 1996). The considered judgments reflected in past decisions constitute relatively fixed points that can be revised only with careful deliberation and good reasons. Overall, there is a commitment to coherence in the giving of reasons—decisions must fit with each other in a plausible reason- and principle-mediated way. Through its reasoning about specific limit-setting decisions, an institution exhibits its moral commitments in an open and educative manner.

A commitment to the transparency that case law requires improves the quality of decision-making. An organization that requires itself to articulate explicit reasons for its decisions becomes more focused in its decision-making deliberations. It might, for example, develop a checklist of key features of coverage decisions, such as the specifications of patient selection criteria and their relevant reasons, including the limits of evidence from clinical trials or the range of patients for whom risk-benefit ratios are acceptable. This kind of explicitness makes it easier for a committee deliberating about coverage to notice the relationship between one decision and others it has made or will have to make. Committee members may become more sensitive to the ways in which the reasons or principles they invoke sometimes conflict. Then they must engage in a difficult deliberation about how to resolve their conflicts and articulate the reasons for a particular resolution.[5]

The disciplined search for coherent reasons embodied in such a case law approach leads to fairer decisions over time for two reasons. First, formal requirements of fairness are better met since public clarity about rationales will promote consistent treatment of similar cases. Second, the discipline involved in specifying the appropriate reasons and making sure they really bear on the case promotes thoughtful evaluation of these reasons and their foundations within our thinking. To the extent that decision makers are then better able to discover flaws in their moral reasoning, they are more likely to arrive at fair decisions. None of this is as likely to happen without a commitment to going public with the rationales for decisions and policies.

If the process improves the fairness of decisions formally and substantively, over time, people will understand better the moral commitments of the institutions making them. If an institution is committed to arriving at fair decisions in a publicly accountable way, we can expect that people will come to recognize this commitment and will see the institution as acting (more) fairly. Only by being explicit about reasons will it be possible for health plans or public agencies to demonstrate that the solutions they adopt for coverage under resource constraints reflect a pattern of reasons and principles that all affected by those decisions should take seriously.

Objections to Reason-Giving

Fear of litigation and exposure in the media are the most commonly expressed objections to our proposal that organizations be more explicit and accountable about the reasons underlying their limit-setting decisions regarding new technologies. Specifically, organizations were concerned that being explicit about reasons would "open the door to attack" from dissatisfied patients and their lawyers or reporters. In part, the fear was that the organization would be exposing the jugular vein of its policies by laying out the grounds for its defense, thereby making itself vulnerable to rebuttal by expert witnesses or to "gaming" (stating falsely that the conditions of coverage have been met) regarding insurance coverage.

The objection and any reply to it both suffer from being speculative. There is simply no evidence that failing to provide reasons for limit-setting decisions protects an organization against litigation or that providing them opens it up to more, or more successful, litigation. Nor is there evidence that disseminating these reasons makes an organization more vulnerable to exposure to bad press. We contend, in fact, that the courts will be less likely to want to substitute their substantive decisions regarding the provision of new technologies if they see health plans or public agencies use robust, careful, deliberative procedures and base their conclusions on reasonable arguments that appeal to the evidence produced in the evaluative process. The best defense against the charge that the organization is negligent in providing contractually promised care is to show that the reasons for limiting access to that care are weighty and justifiable and that decisions were actually based on them. We have some evidence from other kinds of cases, including termination of treatment decisions involving careful ethical reflection, that courts will defer to developed procedures used in medical contexts. Since the courts are notoriously bad places in which to carry out technical assessments of evidence, the courts themselves have good reason not to intrude themselves into decisions about which technologies and treatments have met some reasonable standard of evidence regarding their safety, efficacy, and medical appropriateness.

At the level of the individual clinician, the commonest objection to our emphasis on reason-giving is that busy professionals do not have the time, inclination, or skill to meet this new expectation. This is a serious concern. If accountability for reasonableness means loading extensive burdens on health professionals, it cannot work.

Our response to this concern about overloading busy clinicians is twofold. First, we picture the major new demands as occurring at the level of more forthright political discourse and more forthcoming communication from health plans. We know from our fieldwork that many organizations already deliberate about how to provide the best care for individuals in the context of reasonable resource constraints for a larger population. For these organizations, the only new requirement involves communicating with members and the public in a new, educative way. We do not expect individual clinicians to do this job for the organization.

However, we also envision a learning curve for clinicians over the course of many years, even decades, involving new skills for talking about limits while preserving trust. Early efforts to do this have begun (Pearson, 2000). The change in the way clinicians communicate with their patients about terminal illness and end-of-life concerns shows that, given adequate time for new learning, the kind of change we envision can occur.

We know from conversations with colleagues who support the implicit rationing position that they agree in principle that openness is the desirable approach. They base their opposition to our call for a broad expectation of openness on their conclusion that the costs of openness outweigh the benefits greater openness might provide. The fear underlying their position is that increased openness about limit-setting decisions and policies will increase distrust of doctors and the health care system itself and will lead to more—or more successful—litigation. This is an empirical claim, but since we lack real evidence, it is only speculation. Our view is that, as health plans begin to address the legitimacy and fairness problems by demonstrating that they base limit-setting decisions on a concern for meeting the needs of patients in a covered population under reasonable resource constraints (our Publicity and Relevance Conditions), trust will increase, and litigation—if anything—will go down. Our empirical claim is also speculative, but since the current approach does not work to the satisfaction of anyone, we believe greater openness is the better strategy.

But beyond our belief that greater openness, at worst, is no more likely than our current approach to cause further erosion of trust and increased litigiousness, we see a stronger reason for endorsing accountability for reasonableness. Not giving health plan members and other stakeholders opportunity to understand how and why limits are being set deprives them of an opportunity for participating in a fundamental piece of social governance—the allocation and rationing of services so important for a fundamental human good. Transparency has the potential for enhancing democratic process by helping our society learn how to deal more thoughtfully and fairly with health care resource allocation, a topic we come back to in the final chapter.

CONSTRAINTS ON RATIONALES

The second condition imposes two important constraints on the rationales that can be used to argue for the reasonableness of a limit-setting decision. Specifically, the rationales for coverage decisions should aim to provide (a) a *reasonable* construal of (b) how the organization (or public agency) seeks to provide "value for money" in meeting the varied health needs of a defined population under reasonable resource constraints. Both constraints need explanation.

We may think of the goal of meeting the varied needs of the population of patients under reasonable resource constraints as a characterization of the *common* or *public good* pursued by all engaged in the enterprise of delivering and receiving this care. This goal is avowed in mission statements and medical management philosophy by many health plans, whether they are for-profit or not. It is avowed by clinicians engaged in treatment, who have professional obligations to pursue their patients' best interests. Finally, it is avowed by patients seeking care, who, as long as they are confident that their own needs will be addressed, also want a cooperative scheme that provides affordable, nonwasteful care.

It is not enough simply to specify the goal of the cooperative enterprise. Reasoning about that goal must also meet certain conditions. Specifically, a construal of the goal will be "reasonable" only if it appeals to reasons, including values and principles, that are accepted as relevant by people who are disposed to finding ways of cooperating with each other on mutually acceptable terms. We need to see why this further constraint on reasoning is necessary to be more specific about what it means.

We can begin by asking why reason-giving is appropriate or even demanded in some legal contexts but not others. For example, no reasons are given when juries give verdicts, when state supreme courts refuse review, when trial judges rule on objections, or zoning authorities refuse to grant variances. In his discussion of this question [the examples are his], Harvard Law Professor Frederick Schauer (1995, p. 658) notes that giving reasons (viewed as general rules under which cases are subsumed) is a way to show respect for persons and to "open a conversation" rather than to forestall one:

> Announcing an outcome without giving a reason is consistent with the exercise of authority, for such an announcement effectively indicates that neither discussion nor objection will be tolerated. When the source of a decision rather than the reason behind it compels obedience, there is less warrant for explaining the basis for the decision to those who are subject to it. But when decision makers expect voluntary compliance, or when they expect respect for decisions because the decisions are right rather than because they emanate from an authoritative source, then giving reasons becomes a way to bring the subject of the decision into the enterprise.

Since health plans cannot claim to be an authoritative source—their legitimacy and the fairness of their decision-making is exactly what is at issue—to achieve acceptance and compliance, they "must bring the subject of the decision into the enterprise." The "conversation" the health plan has must be with stakeholders who have diverse moral perspectives on the issues under discussion. Consequently, the giving of reasons must itself respect the moral diversity of those affected by the decisions. Not just any kind of moral reason, compelling as it might be to the decision maker (or the patient) will command recognition of its appropriateness or relevance from those affected by the decision. The reasons offered by decision makers must be those that persons affected by the decisions can recognize as relevant and appropriate.

How the Constraints Limit Reasons

Perhaps the most widely used criteria for technology assessment by health plans are those adopted by the Blue Cross/Blue Shield Medical Advisory Panel (MAP). They require that: *a)* the technology must have final approval from the appropriate government regulatory body; *b)* the scientific evidence must permit conclusions concerning the effect of the technology on health outcomes; *c)* the technology must improve net health outcomes; *d)* it must be as beneficial as any established alternative; and *e)* the improvement must be attainable outside investigational settings. Similar criteria are used by other commercial technology assessment organizations and many individual health plans.

Each of the criteria involves a publicly accessible method of reasoning. Thus, it is easy to establish that a technology has final approval from appropriate regulatory bodies or to establish that controlled clinical trials have been run and show some net health benefit. Adequately trained reviewers can usually agree on the quality of the evidence produced by the available studies or expert panels.[6] Showing that the treatment involves a net benefit to patients and that there is at least as much net benefit as an alternative therapy also involves publicly accessible methods of reasoning, though some further elements of judgment that include evaluation are also involved. There might be some disagreement, for example, about the relative importance of the benefits and risks that attend the treatment, but then it will be clear just what is at issue. Nevertheless, these criteria are ones that all stakeholders should accept as relevant and appropriate—if not sufficient—for making decisions about the inclusion of new technologies in benefit packages. (They may not, in fact, be sufficient since they do not consider costs or cost-effectiveness, which are crucial when decisions are made under strict budget constraints.)

To see their appropriateness more clearly, contrast these criteria with a reason that a religious patient (or clinician) might offer to justify a claim that a treatment be covered. Imagine that her religion requires her to pursue every avenue for survival and that some technology that fails to meet the MAP criteria nevertheless might turn out, she believes, to be the occasion for a miraculous cure. Compelling though this reasoning might be to the patient, it has no relevance at all for those who lack the appropriate faith. The patient (or clinician) advancing it must recognize that she cannot expect those who do not share her faith to give weight to this type of reason or to consider it at all relevant to the deliberation. In contrast, even this religious patient—as opposed, say, to a Christian Scientist—will recognize the relevance of the MAP criteria that bear on establishing the net benefit of the treatment. She is seeking a form of justification that all involved can see is relevant to the common good they pursue: the meeting of patient needs under resource constraints. People whose religious beliefs preclude pursuit of standard medical treatments would not be involved in offering or seeking justification about the inclusion of treatments within the benefit package. They would avoid the cooperative endeavor altogether.

This appeal to the miraculous should be distinguished from disagreements about how to address uncertainty, as in the moral controversy regarding "last-chance" therapies that we discuss in more detail in the next chapter. There is more than one "reasonable" way to manage uncertainty, reflecting more than one way of weighing the importance of the stewardship of scarce resources, the generation of new knowledge through research, and the meeting of urgent patient needs. Consequently, as we argue in the next chapter, health plans might decide these matters differently and yet each be fair in what it concludes.

In our discussion of the importance of reason-giving (required by the Publicity Condition), we argued that a health plan deciding to cover growth hormone treatment only for patients with growth hormone deficiency should provide an explicit rationale for that decision. In that case, the rationale restricts the goal of meeting patients' needs to the treatment of disease and disability and excludes the enhancement of otherwise normal conditions. This reason for excluding some therapies and limiting the use of others is controversial (Daniels, 1996; Daniels, 1992; Buchanan, Brock, Daniels & Wikler, 2000). Many may accept it as characterizing a reasonable limit on the goals of medical coverage, but others may argue that the goals of medical treatment should be broader. For example, they might think that "normal" conditions still impose some competitive disadvantage, and if we have medical interventions that could ameliorate these disadvantages, we should use them. They would argue that if treatment of disease and disability are justified on the basis of protecting opportunity, we should be prepared to cover the use of growth hormone for a disadvantageous condition like extreme shortness, even if the shortness appears to be a normal variation.

Still, proponents on both sides of this dispute can recognize that reasonable people might disagree about the specific requirements of a principle protecting opportunity. Both sides of the dispute about the scope of the goals of medicine nevertheless should recognize the relevance and appropriateness of the kind of reason offered by the other, even if they disagree with the interpretation of the principle or the applications to which it is put.

Once health plans begin to make comparative decisions about technologies and treatments, the perception that the decision-making process produces winners and losers will become clearer. (Comparative decisions, such as those made under budget constraints, involve decisions that meeting the needs of one set of patients is more important than meeting those of others.) Patients who need treatments for which coverage is denied will legitimately complain that they are made worse off by the decision than others whose coverage decisions were favorable. What weight should we give to patients' complaints that they are made worse off than other patients by an unfavorable decision?

Clearly, any decision to cover a treatment benefits some people, just as any decision to exclude a treatment from coverage disadvantages other people (unless the treatment would have been harmful to use). Every comparative decision will make some people better off and some worse off than they would be as a result of some other set of coverage decisions. Because comparative coverage decisions always advantage some and disadvantage others, mere advantage or disadvantage is not a relevant reason in debates about coverage.

There are, however, two sorts of reasons concerning relative advantage or disadvantage that all should consider relevant. First, if a coverage decision disadvantages one patient more than others who are similar in all relevant ways, the decision violates the formal requirement of justice that similar cases be treated similarly. Here the reasoning points to morally objectionable arbitrariness in the outcome. In contrast, if the decision involves an appeal to, say, a lottery for purposes of patient selection, then there is a relevant difference in the winners and losers, namely, that they won or lost the lottery.

Second, if a coverage decision disadvantages someone (and others like him) more than anyone need be disadvantaged under available alternatives, then this too is a reason that all should consider relevant. Whereas the mere fact of being disadvantaged relative to others is a necessary feature of these situations, being disadvantaged more than anyone need be is not. It is the basis for a complaint that each person would want to be able to make were they to turn out to be the person so severely disadvantaged. Therefore, it is a reason that meets the constraints of the Relevance Condition.

The Case of Costs: Cost Effectiveness

How should we view as a reason for excluding coverage the claim that a treatment "costs too much"?

A first point to note, surprising in the context of current distrust of health plans, is that our field work showed that, as of the late 1990s, there was relatively little explicit discussion of costs in the context of technology assessment (as opposed to drug formulary decisions, where costs are more explicitly considered).[7] Costs (or cost-effectiveness) are not included in the Blue Cross/Blue Shield criteria. Of course, a concern about overall magnitude of costs is likely to put a new technology on the agenda of an organization, but the decision-making process we observed involved little explicit discussion of costs. We even saw expert panels avoid explicit requests to consider costs relative to benefits (for example, in evaluating lung volume reduction surgery for chronic pulmonary disease), and we saw one committee decide to provide coverage for a very expensive drug (alglucerase) even to those not covered by a drug benefit.

There are strong reasons for health plans to be leery of claiming that a beneficial technology is too costly in the current climate of public distrust. Saying that a new technology is too costly invites a demand for clarification, both internally to patients and clinicians and externally to would-be enrollees and the public at large. Some clarifications would be widely acceptable, but many others would not. For example, if there were an alternative technology for treating the same condition that had comparable net medical benefits but was less expensive, then being too costly should readily be accepted as a reason for rejecting the more expensive one. Presumably, all would accept avoiding unnecessary costs as a relevant reason.

Outside that simple case—same outcomes at lower cost—clarification of the claim that some technology is too expensive begins to enter controversial terrain. For example, if slightly greater net benefits were possible, especially in the form of decreased risk of death, but only with a much greater cost, there is considerable risk to being criticized for putting so direct a price on the value of life. The case of streptokinase and Tissue-type Plasminogen Activator (TPA), used in dissolving clots in emergency treatment of coronary infarcts, is relevant. The much more expensive drug (TPA) also has only slightly better outcomes, making it quite expensive to acquire the marginal benefit. In the early 1990s, it was demonstrated that the more expensive drug was more widely used in the United States than in Canada, where it was deemed cost-ineffective.

Though properly conducted cost-effectiveness studies of variants on treating the same condition are difficult to perform, health plans might use them were they available. Unfortunately, good studies are expensive and time-consuming to do, and their validity is restricted to the assumptions built into the study, which are often quite specific. So far, with the exception of some minor use of cost-effectiveness studies comparing drugs in the same category, health plans and insurers in the United States have not made much use of this methodology. Health plans and insurers would have less use for "league tables" that rank the cost-effectiveness of treatments for very different conditions. To date this kind of comparative decision-making is not employed by most U.S. insurers, and were it to be used, it would probably be applied only to identify extreme examples of very cost-worthy or cost-unworthy treatments. Used to make finer distinctions, the methodology carries with it the distributive concerns that we discussed in Chapter 3.

A common sentiment revealed in interviews with medical directors and managers of health plans, especially those involved in technology assessment, is that deciding when the medical benefit a technology produces is not cost worthy is a societal, not simply a health plan, decision. Similarly, making comparative decisions across technologies that treat different conditions would also involve judgments that they view as societal, not simply organizational. In the absence of some social consensus, perhaps the result of a public commission charged with making such decisions, health plans are leery of being charged with explicit rationing of new, beneficial technologies, and they are especially leery of being the first on their block to do so. Nor do they relish the idea of defending such a decision in the courts.

Ironically, one of the bugaboos underlying opposition to national health care reform was that it would lead to national agencies making rationing decisions. Better, some insisted, to leave rationing to the implicit workings of the market. But organizations working in that market fear being labeled as rationers if they make the required hard choices. As a result, comparative decision-making about technologies and treatments is currently done much less than the Market Hawks had hoped for. The result is the continued rapid dissemination of technologies and treatments and escalating costs, which will ultimately make the need for comparative decision-making and rationing greater.[8]

Despite the fact that health plans do not make widespread appeals to relative cost-effectiveness or to opportunity costs, such reasons, appropriately supported, would meet the Relevance Condition. If people share in the goal of meeting the varied medical needs of a population covered by limited resources, as well as a commitment to justifying limitations by reference to reasons all can consider appropriate and relevant, then they would be interested in a reason that said a particular intervention had fallen below some defensible threshold of cost-effectiveness or relative cost-worthiness. Not meeting the needs of those for whom the only treatment was marginally effective but quite costly would not be making the affected population of patients worse off than anyone need be, for under reasonable constraints on resources, there will always be some patients whose conditions have no cost-worthy treatment. The burden, in these cases, is to establish the factual presuppositions that underlie giving such a reason. A health plan (or public agency) has to show that its resources are limited in a reasonable way, that the costs and effects are as claimed, that the comparison class of competing interventions it would approve all are superior in the ways claimed, and that there are no special reasons of distributive fairness that override these considerations.

The Case of Costs: Competitive Markets

A health plan might also justify a claim that an intervention is too costly in a very different way—by reference to the competitive economic situation of the health plan. A for-profit plan might argue that to remain competitive it had to provide a reasonable return to investors. A not-for-profit plan might argue that it had to create a reasonable surplus to have the capital it needs for future success. A plan might even argue that the high executive salaries that have attracted public criticism are needed to attract the talented leadership needed to keep the organization competitive. What does accountability for reasonableness say about reasons of this kind?

The answer to this question is complex. To support reasons that refer in this way to the competitive position of the health plan would require providing information that health plans are generally not willing to reveal for quite defensible business reasons. Similarly, supporting arguments for those reasons would often depend on economic and strategic judgments that require special experience and training to make. Ultimately, however, reasons of this kind depend for their credibility on a deeply held but contested belief about the design of current U.S. health care system—the belief that market competition will lead to efficiencies that will work to the advantage of all who have medical needs.

Our point is not that these reasons, in principle, cannot be supported, but that providing support for them requires information that is generally not available, that is hard to understand when it is available, and that ultimately depends on fundamental moral and political judgments about the feasibility of quite different alternative systems for delivering health care. These are deeply contested issues. As a result, appeals to these reasons are likely to fuel further disagreement, not resolve it. By itself, this consequence is not sufficient to reject these kinds of reasons in light of the Relevance Condition. Instead, it shows that we may find ourselves with intractable disagreements about whether the kinds of reasons being advanced are in principle relevant and appropriate. That is part of what we hoped could be avoided by introducing the Relevance Condition, so this is not a welcome outcome. Not surprisingly, health plans have been reluctant to use reasons of this kind to justify limit-setting decisions and policies. In all probability, their reluctance to do so—combined with public suspicion that competitive market factors are often the "real" reason for limits—has contributed to the backlash against the current U.S. health care system itself.

When public disagreement—including disagreement about limits—involves important values, fair process requires a *deliberative* conception of democracy, not a purely procedural appeal to majority rule (see Chapter 3, "Majority Rule" and Fair Process, for a discussion of deliberative democracy). The reasons that play a role in deliberation must be ones that people find acceptable; in this case, this means reasons they find relevant to the problem of meeting health care needs fairly. That is exactly what the Relevance Condition requires.

DISPUTE RESOLUTION PROCEDURES
(REVISION AND APPEALS)

How may a decision concerning coverage of an intervention be challenged by those affected by it? How can a faulty policy be improved? Typically, internal dispute resolution procedures in health plans range from informal complaints to ombudsmen, to more formal grievance procedures with well-defined stages of appeal, to final appeals to panels of medical directors or other last-step internal procedures. Where these mechanisms fail, patients, and even practitioners, may choose to use the threat of litigation or legislative remedies to their complaints. Because these external routes are costly to health plans, it is in their interest to provide for effective internal mechanisms. In fact, National Committee on Quality Assurance (NCQA) standards require health plans to establish appeals and dispute resolution mechanisms.

Dispute resolution procedures in health plans and public agencies play two distinctive roles. Internally, within the health plan or agency, these procedures give members and clinicians an opportunity to voice their perspectives. The procedures create the potential for altered and improved decisions. Externally, these procedures contribute to a wider societal learning curve about the need for limits and the ways in which limits can be set fairly.

Internally, the Revision and Appeals Condition closes the loop between decision makers and those who are affected by their policies. Done well, it engages a broader segment of stakeholders in the process of deliberation. Through these mechanisms, parties that may not have participated in the original decision-making process, and whose views may not have been clearly heard or understood, find a voice, even if after the original fact.

Because the reasons involved in the original decision are publicly accessible (the Publicity Condition) and because decisions are constrained to focus in a reasonable way on meeting the health needs of the insured population under resource constraints (the Relevance Condition), people using the Revision and Appeals Condition to challenge a decision are able to understand the basis on which the decision was made. Even if they did not participate in the original deliberation, the Publicity and Relevance Conditions empower them to reopen the process in the most effective manner.

Of course, this does not mean that every challenge leads to a reconsideration of the decision by the original group responsible for it. It does, however, mean that good arguments that plausibly challenge the original decision are provided a visible and public route back into the policy formulation process. The health plan (or public agency) decision-making process is thus enriched by the new resources for argument the grievance process brings to bear. Conversely, those affected adversely by the original decision are compelled to engage in the process of constrained reason-giving that informed the original decision. Whether specific decisions are actually changed or not, if the arguments raised by these appeals lead to honest reconsideration of the original decision on its merits, they have an important effect on the overall legitimacy of the decision-making process and on its likelihood of achieving fair outcomes. This task plays an educative role for all involved. That is, the appeals and reconsiderations become part of the process through which the broader social deliberation about the problem of limits takes place. The mechanism enables and enhances that broader social process and contributes to the improvement of quality.

A well-developed internal dispute resolution mechanism might reduce the degree to which patients or clinicians adversely affected by decisions seek external authorities or institutions to pursue their interests. Even if litigation or legislation are pursued, however, the fact that there is a robust internal dispute-resolution mechanism can lead to improved external deliberation. This is especially true if the courts come to expect a robust internal mechanism and take up issues only when there is reason to think internal mechanisms have failed in some way.

The courts are ill-equipped to deliberate about the issues of limit setting, especially about the more technical matters involved in assessing efficacy and safety. Court procedures, for example, bring opposing experts to bear, and they leave the final decision up to those—whether judges or juries—with no expertise about technical matters and little understanding of the organizational context within which the issue has arisen. This is simply not be the best way to deliberate about these matters, despite its appearance of a democratic input through the opinion of peers. If, however, a healthy deliberative process, including an exchange of reasons and information in the grievance process, has already taken place, then a court deliberation about the matter may itself involve better deliberation about the merits.

Externally, the Revision and Appeals Condition contributes to a broader social deliberation about the problem of limits and ultimately to democratic governance of health care itself. Even if enrollees and clinicians do not participate in the original decision-making about limits, the Revision and Appeals Condition empowers them to play a more effective role in the larger societal deliberation about the issues. If stakeholders are not satisfied by the internal process, they can turn, in a better informed way, to public institutions that play a role in regulating health plans. By creating the potential for connecting the deliberation that occurs within health plans to wider societal oversight of the limit-setting process, the four conditions we describe play a role in assuring broader accountability of private organizations to those who are affected by limit-setting decisions.

Our position has a bearing on the health reform proposals in the United States that would subject health plans, and not just physicians, to malpractice litigation. Though we are not in principle opposed to this extension of malpractice litigation, it would not substitute for accountability for reasonableness. The four conditions we argue for here are proactive: they are designed to improve patient and population-centered decision-making, not to respond to perceived violations of standards of care. They aim at promoting education about the importance of limits and deliberation about how to set limits fairly, not at erecting legal defenses that may in practice ignore the general problem of meeting needs fairly under resource constraints. Whether or not the extension of malpractice is a good policy move, it would be best implemented only in the context of meeting the four conditions we advocate.

VOLUNTARY OR PUBLIC REGULATION

There are private regulatory mechanisms that conceivably might suffice to ensure that health plans abide by the constraints involved in the Publicity, Relevance, and Revision Conditions. For example, NCQA standards currently require that organizations have procedures for assessing new technologies. These standards, however, do not specify what features the process of technology assessment should have, and they specifically do not include the full transparency about rationales and constraints on reasons that we advocate. If the Publicity, Relevance, and Revision Conditions were fully incorporated into NCQA standards, an important private regulatory process would come into play. Employers and others seeking to do business only with accredited health plans would be assured they were doing business with organizations that had incorporated steps toward addressing the fairness and legitimacy problems health plans now face.

Failure to adopt the Publicity, Relevance, and Revision Conditions voluntarily, or through the nonlegal coercive force of sanctions from private associations, could set the stage for public regulation. At the end of the 1990s, many state legislatures were already deliberating about, or passing regulations governing, the behavior of health plans and other insurers, including restrictions on "gag" orders or other constraints on what physicians may say to patients and often, provision for appeals procedures. Our analysis of how to solve the legitimacy and fairness problems is neutral between public regulation and voluntary private enforcement of the conditions we outline, though we believe that, ultimately, public regulation will be required. In theory, either would suffice to establish the kind of accountability that is necessary where fundamental issues of fairness are involved, provided that the process meets our four conditions. In theory, either can facilitate a broader public

rals and to include room for "medically necessary" exceptions in pharmacy benefit restrictions—all go beyond simple market accountability and involve appeals
to the reasonableness of restrictions. For example, market accountability alone
would only require that health plans inform us of their emergency room coverage
policies. Accountability for reasonableness, however, would endorse the requirement that health plans reimburse emergency room visits when a prudent or reasonable lay person sought emergency services for a condition that any such person would view as highly risky to health or life.

In the next six chapters we explore in more detail what accountability for reasonableness means in the context of health plan or public agency decisions to set
limits about last-chance therapies (Chapter 5); coverage for new procedures like
lung volume reduction surgery (Chapter 6); and pharmacy benefits (Chapter 7).
We also explore what the four conditions mean for policies of indirect limit setting that depend on giving incentives to clinicians to reduce or modify the utilization of medical services (Chapter 8) and in the context of contracting by public
purchasers for mental health services (Chapter 9). Finally, we briefly explore how
the experience in several developed and developing countries contribute to a social learning curve about setting limits fairly (Chapter 10).

The examples of accountability for reasonableness in action presented in Chapters 5–10 do not provide algorithms that will solve thorny questions about resource allocation. Accountability for reasonableness does not offer new reasons or
rules for decision makers to apply in seeking fair health care limits. The bad news
is that there is often more than one defendable answer to real-world questions
about health care limits.

The good news, however, is that the range of reasonable answers is limited, and
accountability for reasonableness can help us narrow the range. Chapters 5–9 will
illustrate how the four conditions help health plans and public agencies deal with
specific areas of limit setting. Over time, recurrent deliberations add to an organization's (and society's) "case law." This process can build consensus about relevant reasons, simplify new limit-setting questions, and promote better decisions
and policies.

As organizations, agencies, and the public gain experience with setting limits
fairly, each new question will not require the equivalent of lifting ourselves by our
bootstraps. Even in the absence of any widely acceptable principles that would
deductively yield one—and only one—answer to questions about limits, accountability for reasonableness allows organizations and society itself to increase its skill
at reaching justifiable conclusions.

NOTES

1. The coalition included Kaiser Permanente, Group Health Cooperative of Puget Sound,
HIP Health Insurance, the American Association of Retired Persons, and Families USA.

2. These conditions were developed independently but fit reasonably well with the principles of publicity, reciprocity, and accountability governing democratic deliberation cited by Amy Gutmann and Dennis Thompson (1996). For reservations about their account, see Daniels (1999).

3. When Harvard Pilgrim Health Care, one of our collaborators in the work we report on in later chapters, was put into receivership during 2000, confidence in the integrity of the organization was crucial to its survival. Its experience suggests that accountability for reasonableness would increase public perception of the integrity of those organizations whose decisions show commitment to promoting population health fairly.

4. A broader study showed some variation in insurance practices, however (Finklestein, Silvers & Marrero, 1998; Sabin & Daniels, 1998).

5. Schauer (1995, p. 657) notes that "decision makers themselves are unlikely to fully apprehend and appreciate this function [that reason-giving increases discipline], for most decision makers underestimate the need for external quality control of their own decisions. But when institutional designers have grounds for believing that decisions will systematically be the product of bias, self-interest, insufficient reflection, or simply excess haste, requiring decision makers to give reasons may counteract some of these tendencies."

6. When we discuss the decisions made around bone marrow transplants for advanced breast cancer in Chapter 5, however, we can see that there was some disagreement about whether these criteria were actually satisfied in a particular case.

7. Kaiser Permanente received national attention because its decision not to cover Viagra for members was explicitly based on concerns about costs.

8. The problem has the structure of what game theorists call a many-person prisoner's dilemma (Daniels, 1988).

9. If organizations that put reasons forward (call them "icebreakers") actually benefited, then the coordination problem we describe comes from a misestimate of what self-interested action calls for. It is the misestimate that sets up the public goods problem (the "many person prisoners" dilemma) informally described in the text. If organizations that act as icebreakers when others fail to do so actually do worse, then we have a true "many persons prisoners" dilemma.

5

MANAGING LAST-CHANCE THERAPIES

The most difficult and explosive responsibility for any health care system is deciding whether patients with life-threatening illnesses will receive insurance coverage for unproven treatments they believe may make the difference between life and death.

Potentially life-saving treatments with proven efficacy and safety (proven net benefit), and quack treatments for which there is no scientific rationale, rarely pose major problems about insurance coverage. In a country as wealthy as the United States, effective last-chance treatments without alternatives generally are and should be covered virtually all the time. When shared resources from cooperative schemes are involved, as in public or private insurance, rather than individuals paying with their own resources, quack treatments will and should virtually never be covered, even if the patient or doctor passionately believe in the purported cure.

The difficult practical and ethical challenges come from promising but unproven last-chance treatments, for which we use high-dose chemotherapy with autologous bone marrow transplant (ABMT) for advanced breast cancer as our key example.[1] Not covering treatments that ultimately prove to be effective lets curable patients die prematurely, and even if a treatment ultimately proves to be ineffective, not covering it may create the impression that critically ill patients are being abandoned in their moment of need. Covering treatments that ultimately prove to be ineffective or harmful reduces the quantity and quality of the patient's remaining life, wastes substantial resources, and undermines clinical research. These are the moral stakes in the decision.

There are also other costs and risks in these decisions. Denials of coverage for seriously ill people are highly visible. Even health plans that use impeccable science and patient-centered deliberation while trying to hold the traditional, contractually specified, line against unproven therapies risk horrendous publicity, expensive litigation, and legislative mandates requiring coverage. Visibility for denials of last-chance therapies also plagues public agencies, a point to which we return in more detail later.

There is room for reasonable people to disagree about how to weigh the conflicting values and principles in these cases. There is no convincing, principled argument or social consensus for determining the relative importance of *1)* giving some (how much?) priority to meeting the urgent claims of patients in last-chance situations, *2)* providing stewardship of collective resources, *3)* producing the public good of scientific knowledge about the effectiveness of unproven therapies, and *4)* respecting patient autonomy through collaborative decision-making about risks and benefits.

We can try to gloss over the ethical uncertainties in these cases by pretending that terms like "investigational," "experimental," and "medical necessity" tell us what to do. These terms, however, explain little and dodge the genuine ethical dilemmas. Without extensive explanation of the reasoning process they will not, and should not, satisfy the public or the courts. The ethical challenges posed by unproven but promising last-chance technologies are not helped at all by the language of current medical insurance benefit contracts in the United States. They are also made harder to solve by the climate of distrust that surrounds insurers, including health plans of all types.

We return to a version of our central question: Under what conditions should the public accept as *legitimate* and *fair,* decisions made by health plans or public agencies that limit access to "unproven" last-chance therapies, especially if some responsible clinicians and their patients believe them to be effective?

In answering this question, we draw on results from a three-year research project involving collaboration with a number of leading managed care organizations. Through a series of policy case studies, we have been investigating how insurers and health plans make coverage decisions about the adoption and application of new technologies—the visible tip of the limit-setting iceberg. We report in this chapter on some very promising exemplary practices we have observed for managing last-chance therapies. Each of these practices illustrates accountability for reasonableness. We believe it would be premature to try to choose among these exemplary practices. Because of the deep moral disagreement about the underlying issues, it would be wise for society to experiment with several promising strategies in order to learn more over time about how well they work and how morally acceptable they seem in light of actual practice.

Before describing the moral disagreement further and the exemplary practices we observed, we begin with some background about the scientific and societal context in which the practices we describe have developed.

A BRIEF SOCIAL HISTORY

By 1990, patients with advanced breast cancer, with the support of some clinicians, began to seek coverage for admittedly experimental use of ABMT from health plans, including our collaborating sites. In this treatment, patients are given very large doses of chemotherapy, in the hope that the massive chemical attack on the cancer will eliminate it. Because the chemotherapy also destroys the patient's blood-forming bone marrow, the patient's marrow is removed before the procedure and then reinfused after the chemotherapy. Analogues to this treatment had proven effective for some lymphatic cancers, and there was some scientific rationale for extending the treatment to solid tumors. Despite the enthusiasm of the clinicians and the desperate hope of the breast cancer patients, many of whom were well organized and informed, there was at the time no hard clinical evidence, and especially no controlled trials, that showed an advantage to the risky treatment over standard treatments.

During this period in the early 1990s, technology assessment of the therapy was undertaken at a number of our collaborating health plans and by the Medical Advisory Panel (MAP) of the Blue Cross Blue Shield Technology Evaluation Center (TEC). The National Cancer Institute authorized four randomized clinical trials for ABMT in advanced breast cancer in 1991 (with support from TEC), but these results would not be available until late in the decade. There were no published controlled clinical trials until the Bezwoda study in 1995 (Bezwoda, Seymour & Dansey). Early evaluations of this technology had to be based on weaker forms of evidence. Between 1991 and 1994, several health plans (as well as the Oregon Health Services Commission) decided that the technology was not ready for standard coverage, based on early evidence regarding safety and efficacy. (As early as 1990, one of our collaborating sites, Health Partners, provided coverage under alternative funding for participation in clinical trials.) Similarly, early evaluations by the MAP found that there was inadequate evidence of efficacy or net benefit for ABMT for advanced breast cancer.

It was not until February 1996 that the MAP finally decided that the therapy did meet its criteria for status as a noninvestigational technology. At its February 1996 meeting, the MAP evaluated evidence from the only published study of a randomized clinical trial (Bezwoda, Seymour & Dansey, 1995), as well as evidence from ongoing studies. The discussion suggested that the published study could not support conclusions about the greater efficacy of the therapy over standard treatments used in the United States, but the MAP voted that its criteria were met.[2]

A consideration of the identical evidence in June 1996 by California Blue Shield led to the decision that the MAP criteria were not yet satisfied.[3] Several health plans that had undertaken similar technology assessments also continued to believe, as of mid-1996, that there was insufficient evidence to show that the therapy met reasonable criteria of safety and efficacy for advanced breast cancer in comparison to standard treatments—even if it had by then become nearly standard therapy.

Like HIV patients desperate to try promising drugs prior to full Food and Drug Administration (FDA) testing, however, breast cancer patients in the early 1990s demanded that they be allowed to decide whether the risks were worth taking (Daniels 1995). The gatekeeper for ABMT, however, was not the FDA, charged with keeping unsafe pharmaceuticals off the market, but insurers, who, by contract, had no obligation to provide coverage for investigational treatments. When some managed care organizations (MCO)s, with adequate, evidence-based reason on their side, insisted the therapy was still investigational and unproven, and might even prove worse than standard therapies, patients pursued both litigation and legislation, and the media "exposed" the denials. As early as 1991, *60 Minutes* featured a story about Aetna declining coverage for ABMT for breast cancer. In California in 1993, the estate of Neline Fox won an $89 million suit against Healthnet, which had originally denied coverage, and then provided it. The suit charged the delay cost Fox her life. This suit cast a pall over traditional procedures for assessing the status of last-chance therapies.

Throughout the early 1990s, many insurers were providing coverage for patients participating in approved clinical trials. Unfortunately, this coverage seemed "arbitrary and capricious" according to an important study (Peters & Rogers, 1994) in the *New England Journal of Medicine,* which said coverage was not correlated with pretreatment clinical characteristics of the patients, the design or phase of the study, or the response to induction therapy. That study showed that as many as three out of four patients seeking coverage for participation in a trial were granted it, and another half of those who threatened legal action when initially denied also received coverage. Activism clearly paid off for patients seeking treatment.

Responding to well-organized and highly visible advocates for breast cancer patients, some state legislatures mandated coverage as early as 1994 and 1995, despite protests, for example in Minnesota and Massachusetts, that the mandates would make it impossible to continue proper clinical trials aimed at finding out if the procedure was truly superior to standard therapy. In other states, though legislative mandates were not passed, lawsuits in effect compelled coverage, since large punitive damages were imposed where coverage was denied or delayed. The resulting legal climate made it too risky and costly to deny what was still an unproven therapy.

Some insurers responded earlier than others to the handwriting on the wall, reading the message that traditional efforts to manage last-chance therapies by holding the line against investigational treatments were not working. Following the *60 Minutes* "exposé" in 1991, Aetna, under the initiative of William Mc-Givney, introduced a procedure in which an independent panel would be invoked when patients wanted a last-chance treatment for which an internal review had denied coverage. (We return to this procedure shortly.) The same approach was adopted by Kaiser Permanente of Northern California in 1993. Other approaches were introduced in the same period, including, in 1994, Oregon Blue Cross Blue Shield's use of a transplant coordinator to manage the coverage of clinical trials for unproven last-chance therapies. In 1996, Health Partners introduced a special process for evaluating promising therapies that fell in the space between clearly investigational and standard treatment. It is this new wave of approaches that is the focus of our discussion in subsequent sections.

Before turning to the details of these newer approaches, we want to make four points. First, the social climate—including well-organized women's groups, a crusading media, committed practitioners, suspicious courts, and opportunistic legislators—clearly made the standard "technology assessment" approach to holding the line against coverage for last-chance investigational therapies untenable. Second, the legal and political interventions also had the effect of making it more difficult to find out if high-dose chemotherapy with stem cell support actually worked for advanced breast cancer. Although some MCOs decided to provide coverage for clinical trials, others (for example, Harvard Community Health Plan, in an evaluation just before the Massachusetts mandate in 1994) were ethically uneasy about insisting on participation in trials, where patients would not always get the experimental regimen. The effect of compelling coverage meant that enrollment in NIH-sponsored clinical trials was slowed. The public intervention through the courts and legislatures thus had the effect of frustrating another publicly supported goal in health care, namely, to make the system more efficient by pushing it to adopt "outcomes-based" medicine.

Third, it was not until 1999 that firm evidence from controlled trials became available about the medical benefits of ABMT for advanced breast cancer, and the result makes the story we have been narrating all the more poignant. For all the struggle about this therapy, it turns out to have no significant effect on mortality and may in fact be worse than lower-dose chemotherapy regimens (Stadtmauer, O'Neill, Goldstein et al., 2000). Thus, strategies for managing last-chance therapies that emphasized enrollment in clinical trials have the weight of reason—and hindsight—on their side.

Fourth, the challenge to limit setting by health plans has its international analogues in publicly administered and financed health care systems that offer universal coverage, as we note in Chapter 10. Even where public agencies might be thought to be a more legitimate locus for limit-setting decisions, a similar moral challenge is made. The suggestion is that bureaucratic decisions driven too much by budget limitations ignore the fact of urgent need in these cases; that is, that the moral priorities of decision makers are inappropriate. It is important to see that the moral dimension of these issues arises across differences in institutional design, financing, national culture and even incentives (see Chapter 10).

MORAL DISAGREEMENT AND ACCESS
TO LAST-CHANCE THERAPIES

Reasonable people disagree about the best way to manage access to last-chance therapies because they disagree about the relative importance of several values or principles that come into conflict in these cases. In a pluralist society, where the underlying disagreement may involve conflicts among more comprehensive and systematic moral views, this means there is no one way of managing last-chance therapies that all will agree is morally superior. In effect, we may have to learn to live with alternative best practices, not agreement on one approach, even if (as we discuss later) this raises a challenge to one aspect of our traditional thinking about fairness and justice.

The general and difficult moral problem that all health plans must solve is how to meet the diverse needs of the insured population under reasonable resource constraints. This problem involves balancing population-centered concerns against patient-centered ones. Promising, but unproven, last-chance treatments evoke the general problem especially sharply since so much is at stake for the individual patients, while, at the same time, the proposed treatments are often quite costly.

The major population-centered concerns are the prudent use of shared resources ("stewardship") and the promotion of public goods, such as knowledge about safety and efficacy produced through clinical trials. Those who emphasize these concerns will prefer policies under which collective resources would only be used for last-chance treatments that meet a threshold of established net benefit, and unproven therapies, if paid for at all, would only be covered in the context of controlled clinical trials, including randomized controlled trials in which a patient might receive the standard treatment or a placebo if there is no standard treatment.

The key patient-centered concerns include: giving proper attention to patient needs, especially urgent needs as in the last-chance situations; avoiding harm, including the psychological harm that can arise from adversarialism; supporting hope; and managing uncertainties and risks through collaborative treatment planning. Those who emphasize these concerns will prefer policies for last-chance treatments that create a much lower standard of evidence that must be met for a treatment to be offered to a patient and that allow patients and their clinicians more leeway in judging the relative weight of risks and benefits. They are less likely to promote policies that would require patients to enter controlled trials, since they have no assurance in those trials of receiving the desired treatment.

Reasonable people will differ, however, in the degree to which they want to trade population-centered values in favor of patient-centered ones because of the urgency of the situation. There is no higher-level agreement on how much weight to give to competing values or principles. Careful deliberation may resolve some of the conflicts, for often our views are not systematically considered, but it is unlikely to eliminate all of them. In many cases, the disagreement about how to weigh these values may reflect significant differences in comprehensive moral views that people hold. For example, some communitarians will give more weight to guardianship of collective resources and the maximization of health benefits for a community that is cooperating to share resources than to meeting individually defined needs. Classic liberals will give more weight to respect for individual autonomy than to obligations of stewardship. Both communitarians and liberals will recognize the relevance of the reasons to which the other gives priority, since in other contexts, these factors also count in their thinking about how to solve the general problem of meeting needs under resource constraints. But the disagreement about weights or priorities will probably persist.

This disagreement about weights will then lead people to have different views about the acceptability of different ways of managing last-chance therapies. What is striking about the practices we now describe is the way in which they bring out the importance of deliberation and the transparency of appropriate rationales for the management practice, and the crucial role of open processes for revision and appeals.

SOME EXEMPLARY PRACTICES IN MANAGING
LAST-CHANCE THERAPIES

We begin with the earliest approach to managing last-chance therapies, the terminal illness program William McGivney started at Aetna in 1991. This program, used primarily in an indemnity insurance context, served as Aetna's modus operandi until the end of 1996 after Aetna purchased and merged with US HealthCare. It was later adapted for use in a health-plan setting by Northern California Kaiser Permanente. Eventually, it became the model for the 1996 Friedman-Knowles legislation in California and was proposed in the late 1990s as a component of national health care reform in some versions of the Patients' Bill of Rights.

In the Aetna program, when medical directors in the field received a request for an unproven but promising last-chance cancer treatment that was not covered under established company policy, they referred the request to the home office in

Hartford, Connecticut, where a consulting oncologist reviewed the clinical situation. A key feature of the program was that the consultant was only empowered to *approve* requests. If she believed the request did not represent reasonable clinical practice for the particular patient, the case was automatically referred outside the company for independent review by the Medical Care Ombudsman Program in Bethesda, Maryland.

The Ombudsman Program, founded by Grace Monaco in 1991, provides independent expert opinion about appropriate treatment in serious but ambiguous clinical situations. On a timetable which can be as short as 24 hours, the Ombudsman Program will put together a panel of two-to-three experts, with no affiliation to the insurer or the provider of the proposed treatment, to assess whether the proposed treatment has any scientific rationale for the particular patient. This is not a technology assessment of the new technology but an expert clinical assessment of the potential value of the technology for a particular patient. Typically, at least one of the experts is prepared to testify in court if the case should come to litigation.

Aetna did not restrict its own consulting oncologist from rendering negative coverage decisions because the consultant lacked competence. Any time that specialized technical expertise was needed, Aetna could have hired additional consultants at less cost to itself than using the Ombudsman Program. The problem Aetna was trying to solve with its terminal illness program was one of *trust*, not lack of technical expertise. The fact and appearance of conflict of interest was removed: if Aetna would say no only if an independent consultant said no, then the "no" should not be construed as a cost-driven decision. In circumstances of life-threatening illness and ambiguous information, the patient's trust in the decision-making process can be the difference between peace and outrage, or acceptance versus litigation.

In 1993, the Northern California region of Kaiser Permanente took the program that Aetna had developed in a primarily indemnity insurance context and adapted it for its own 3600-physician prepaid group practice HMO. Kaiser's experience helps us understand the mechanism through which Aetna's innovative way of addressing the patient's concern about the insurer's potential conflict of interest helps the decision-making process (Beebe, Rosenfeld & Collins, 1997).

Like Aetna, Northern California Kaiser Permanente decided to let patients in last-chance situations know that they could go outside of Kaiser for an independent opinion from the Ombudsman Program if they were not satisfied with the internal decision-making process. This was a controversial step for Kaiser to take. Some Kaiser doctors worried that allowing automatic appeal outside the HMO would diminish the group's ability to manage care rationally and feared that the program itself might be very costly.

What actually happened was exactly the opposite of what was feared. From 1994–1996, only six of the 2.5 million northern California members asked for referral to the Ombudsman Program. When the patients' concerns about insurer trustworthiness and potential conflict of interest were addressed in advance by the option of going outside of Kaiser for independent consultation, patients and families were much readier to enter into a reflective dialogue with their Kaiser physicians about what treatment approach really made sense for them.

The Aetna-Kaiser last-chance policy might simply be dismissed as a cost-benefit calculation made by the health plan. Put cynically, it is better to pay for a few treatments than face lawsuits, any one of which would be more costly than a bunch of treatments. But it also can be defended—and is by some MCOs that adopt it—on more explicitly moral grounds that connect its adoption with our earlier discussion of accountability for reasonableness and the four conditions.

The policy can be defended morally in this way: it recognizes the fundamental importance in a medical system of shared decision-making between patients and clinicians about risk taking. If an unproven last-chance therapy is viewed by some acknowledged experts as the most appropriate treatment for the patient, and if the patient understands the risks as presented by parties on all sides, then organizations have no better option than to rely on the informed decision of the patient and her clinician. This is not the same as saying that a patient can be granted any last wish regarding treatment; there must be some basis in evidence and expert view that the therapy is not quackery. In the external review model, that expert view is provided by the independent panel. Under those conditions, simply refusing to provide coverage fails to acknowledge the obligation not to impose paternalistically a plan's own judgment about acceptable risks and benefits on the choices of desperately ill patients with few options. To be sure, the role of the MCO as a guardian of shared resources is reduced, but this is defensible in light of both the urgency of the patients' needs and the special importance, in light of the uncertainty and the severity of need, of promoting a climate of shared decision-making. Indeed, a proponent of this view might even say that the decision to hold to a hard-line denial is so likely to lead to a waste of resources in the legal and political climate that actually surrounds MCOs that the more efficient way to respect resources is to adopt the more lenient strategy toward last-chance therapies.

The Aetna-Kaiser approach has been embodied in recent legislation. Under the Friedman-Knowles Experimental Treatment Act, passed by the California legislature in 1996, the kind of independent consultation process that Aetna and Kaiser Permanente of Northern California provide became mandatory for all California insurers on July 1, 1998. The provisions of the bill are quite detailed, but the basic concept is simple: If a patient with a condition that has no effective therapy and is likely to cause death within two years is denied coverage for a new treatment with some scientific promise, an independent expert review of the decision must be offered.

What is so important about the Friedman-Knowles bill is the effort to use legislation to influence the quality of the decision-making process without making any attempt to mandate what the decisions themselves should be. The bill does not mandate any specific treatments as so many states have done and continue to do. Rather, it mandates an organizational decision-making process designed to reduce fears about conflict of interest and increase deliberative reflection and clarity about the reasons for coverage decisions. In our terms, it promotes accountability for reasonableness.

Oregon Blue Cross Blue Shield developed an approach to unproven bone marrow transplant regimens that reflected a slightly different moral framework. In 1993, in the aftermath of the Fox vs. Healthnet case, Oregon Blue Cross Blue Shield created a new, full-time role of transplant coordinator. The transplant coordinator is a clinically experienced nurse whose job is to work directly with patients and families, transplant programs, employers, and the Oregon Blue Cross Blue Shield benefit systems to create mutually satisfactory individualized treatment plans.

Whereas Aetna and Kaiser use the option for independent review outside of the organization to allay patient concerns about conflict of interest and promote collaboration, Oregon Blue Cross Blue Shield's distinctive approach is an unusually open and accountable process of deliberation and reason-giving with an especially strong emphasis on supporting scientific treatment evaluation. Instead of the infamous "gag rule" (insurance contract restrictions on what physicians could say to insured patients), the Oregon program has developed what might be called a "let's talk it over openly and at great length" rule!

In ethics classes at medical, nursing, and business schools, we try to teach students to identify the key facts and values in a situation and to develop options to advance the most important values that apply. This is what the Blue Cross transplant coordinator does every day, except that she does it under circumstances of time pressure and high emotion, not in a classroom. When we interviewed her for our research project, we told her that her role seemed to be one-third nurse clinician, one-third nurse manager and one-third ethics professor.

Here are the kinds of things the transplant coordinator says in dealing with the multiple stakeholders in the decision-making process:

- To a confused and frightened patient: "Do you have this article about the treatment? Have you read this other one? I'm going to be at the library this afternoon—why don't you come and meet me there and we can go over the information together?"
- To explain the importance of consistency to a wealthy patient: "Just because you're a VIP who lives in the West Hills, you don't really want me to treat you any differently than the person who comes to clean your house, do you?"
- To an employer who wants Blue Cross to cover an employee for a treatment that has no scientific justification: "But it's not based on sound science. Do you want to do the same thing for all the other women in your employee

group? And even if you do, what will you tell their sisters who can't have the treatment? We want to be able to support scientific research that's going to answer the question."

- And, to a provider who is asking the insurer to cover an unproven treatment: "Then build your case to us, make your proposal so that when we make this decision, we can have sound rationale for a similar case on the next patient that you or someone else may send to us."

These comments illustrate the kind of deliberative dialogue that will have to happen hundreds of thousands and perhaps millions of times for doctors, patients, health plans, and society to move along a learning curve towards a more patient-centered, cost-effective, and ethical health care system.

The Oregon Blue Cross Blue Shield process, like the Aetna-Kaiser process, places its ultimate emphasis on encouraging open deliberation between patient, clinician, and, in this case, coordinator. When we asked the coordinator how she was able to achieve trust with patients without the promise of an external, independent review, as in the Aetna-Kaiser approach, she said that she would view an instance of a patient going to external review as a failure on her part to have engaged the patient in the kind of deliberative give-and-take that her approach requires. The promise of external review, she feared, could lure patients away from the need to engage in deliberation with her.

Although deliberation and shared decision-making were the key goals, Oregon Blue Cross Blue Shield has another priority as well—supporting clinically important research. If a promising but unproven last-chance treatment is available in a scientifically valid clinical trial, the plan will cover it. The coordinator reported that no patients had resorted to litigation, and a significant number decided that the unproven treatments they initially requested were, after careful thinking, not really what they wanted.

In contrast to the Aetna-Kaiser approach, Oregon Blue Cross Blue Shield appears to put more emphasis on redirecting its stewardship responsibility toward supporting research. At the same time, since outright denial of unproven therapies is much less likely than in a traditional "hold the line" approach, it becomes possible to involve the patient in shared decision-making.

In 1996, Health Partners, a prominent HMO in Minnesota, began to develop a special policy regarding promising but still unproven therapies. For selected promising treatments, Health Partners will provide coverage, even though the technology still falls into the investigational category and would traditionally be excluded from coverage by contract language. The rationale for singling out the category of promising treatments is to introduce consistent policy about a particular technology, thereby avoiding case-by-case responses to individual requests.

Although this approach clearly relaxes the traditional hard line about stewardship, it keeps the health plan in control of what counts as promising. Compared to the case-by-case decision-making by Aetna, Kaiser of Northern California, and Oregon Blue Cross Blue Shield, the Health Partners approach appears to place more emphasis on the organization's stewardship role. It remains to be seen whether the approach of offering greater consistency technology-by-technology at the cost of less flexibility in deciding individual cases leads to more or less conflict and litigation.

ACCOUNTABILITY FOR REASONABLENESS AND EXEMPLARY PRACTICES

The procedures we have described for managing last-chance therapies can be adapted to the four conditions that constitute accountability for reasonableness. The first point to note is that the rationale for a plan's adopting one procedure rather than another should itself be made public, as the Publicity Condition requires. In such a rationale, giving more weight to responsibility for stewardship (as perhaps in the "promising therapy" strategy) than another strategy does is the type of reason that meets the Relevance Condition; so does the opposite weighting. Our main point is that each of the exemplary strategies could be defended publicly with reasons that meet the legitimacy conditions. What varies among these procedures is not the appeal to inappropriate reasons but the different weights reasonable people might give to relevant reasons.

In their implementation, any of these procedures could meet the other conditions as well. For example, in the procedure followed by Oregon Blue Cross Blue Shield in managing patients who may be left out of available clinical trials, there is an effort to engage the patient in reason-giving of exactly the sort required by the Relevance Condition. Can an appropriate trial be located elsewhere or created? Are there alternative approaches consistent with the values the program is committed to? Does the proposed course of action set a precedent that can be followed in the future? The results of previous deliberations about particular cases could be made publicly available (always respecting confidentiality), so they were accessible to other patients seeking to develop claims about coverage in their own situations. In effect, a kind of case law could emerge that would govern the operation of the health plan and be accessible to patients and clinicians. In similar fashion, the kind of deliberation engaged in by the external ombudsman program used by Aetna and Kaiser, and now mandated by California law, could also meet the publicity conditions and the restrictions on types of reason-giving.

We noted earlier that the legitimacy problem in the United States has its analogue in publicly administered systems. In other countries, even where public commissions have been established to approve principles for priority setting and limit setting within the national system, the agencies that make actual decisions often keep their results quiet, perhaps implicit in quietly made budget decisions, and fail to meet the four conditions of accountability for reasonableness. We believe compliance with these conditions would contribute to establishing greater legitimacy for hard choices made in those systems as well and return to discuss public agencies in more detail in Chapter 10.

FORMAL VS. PROCEDURAL JUSTICE

The examples cited in this chapter suggest that there is not just one best or fairest way to manage last-chance therapies. At least, reasonable people may not agree on what the best procedure is, and in light of that disagreement, we believe that societies should experiment with a family of best practices. There is, however, a troubling implication of this view that some may view as a fatal objection. We see it not as a flaw in our approach but as a manifestation of an unavoidable moral uncertainty, which we must learn to respect and to live with.

Here is the problem: Suppose we have two patients, Groucho and Harpo, who are indistinguishable with regard to the relevant features of their cases. Both make the same claim that they need a particular high-dose chemotherapy with stem cell support for their advanced cancers. Let us suppose that this treatment has not yet been shown to provide a net benefit for the condition, which is, in any case, fatal on standard treatments. Groucho belongs to BestHealth and Harpo to GreatCare, two responsible MCOs that manage last-chance therapies in different ways. For the sake of specificity, suppose BestHealth uses a version of the external appeal procedure (like Aetna or Kaiser) and that GreatCare covers people in clinical trials if they meet the protocols or can make a reasonable case that they should be so covered (like Oregon Blue Cross Blue Shield). Suppose, finally, that Groucho is denied the transplant, but that Harpo is given it. When Groucho hears about Harpo, should we agree if he complains that one of them has been treated unfairly?

Groucho claims that a fundamental principle of justice has been violated, the *formal* principle that like cases be treated similarly. If his case is just like Harpo's in all relevant ways, then they should either both get the treatment or neither should. The formal principle does not tell us how both should be treated, only that they should be treated similarly. Specifically, if there are *reasons* why Harpo should get the treatment, Groucho insists, then they apply equally to him, and he should receive it as well.

Groucho's complaint that a formal principle of justice is violated actually turns on there being a substantive reason or principle that grounds the decision to treat Harpo. To see this point, consider this variation on the case: in both MCOs, a coin is flipped about whether to give the treatment. Groucho loses and Harpo wins. When Groucho complains that like cases are being treated dissimilarly, we can now say to him, "The cases are unlike; there was a coin toss, and you lost and he won." There is no violation of the formal principle if there is a non-reason-based procedure used to distinguish the cases, as there is in the case of a coin toss. Alternatively, we can construe this as a case in which a principle is appealed to and uniformly applied, namely, the principle that winners, but not losers, of coin tosses (or other random processes) will get the treatment.

Neither BestHealth nor GreatCare flips coins, however. Within their different procedures, each encourages giving reasons and deliberating about cases in light of reasons. We presuppose that the difference in their procedures for managing these cases rests on a difference in the weights the two organizations give to certain values, i.e., the values of urgency, stewardship, and shared decision-making with patients. Suppose further that we are right to claim there is no argument we all can accept that shows that one weighting of these values (and thus one procedure) is clearly morally more justifiable than the other. That weighting, and thus the choice of fair procedure, is itself the focus of reasonable disagreement.

Generally, when there is a violation of the formal principle of justice, we are challenged to evaluate the weight attributed to a reason or principle that was applied in one case but not the other. We are asked to find a difference in the cases, that is, to show that they were not really similar in all relevant ways, or to affirm the uniform application of that reason or principle or of some alternative principle. But in the condition of moral pluralism we face, we have no candidate principle that enjoys our endorsement independently of the fair procedure we are employing. A reason that may seem compelling or decisive in one process may not have that force in another. To be sure, we are not flipping coins in either case. We are deliberating carefully in a reason-driven and reason-giving way. But the weight given reasons in each setting is a reasonable reflection of other moral disagreements and moral uncertainty—the very uncertainty about what counts as a just outcome that compels us to adopt a procedural approach to fair outcomes. Groucho can be told this: "Harpo was given the treatment because his plan reasoned about his case differently than your plan, and both ways of reasoning are relevant and arguably fair."

How tolerable would a system be if it produced situations in which a Groucho and Harpo were treated differently? We might think it makes a difference how centralized or decentralized a system is. In a decentralized system such as ours, for example, it may be difficult to require that insurance schemes use one, rather than another, procedurally fair way of deliberating about cases (though legislation such as the Friedman-Knowles Experimental Treatment Act imposes uniformity, at least at one stage of decision-making). On what basis should the choice between procedures and weightings be made? Can we show a superior outcome by insisting on one such process rather than another? Without such a compelling regulatory reason, we might have trouble justifying public regulation requiring just one form of managing last-chance cases.

Despite the decentralization in our health care system, however, our courts arguably can impose a kind of unifying framework. Groucho might sue BestHealth, saying that not only does he want the treatment, and not only does his clinician say it is appropriate, but GreatCare has given the treatment to someone just like him. In practice, the courts could make unworkable an effort to experiment with different fair procedures to see what their advantages and disadvantages really are. On the other hand, what has often carried the day in actual suits on these matters is a demonstration of a lack of fair process and a kind of arbitrariness within an organization. If each of the fair procedures constitutes a reasonable defense against that sort of claim, then the courts might welcome an effort to rely more directly on fair procedures applied within plans. An analogy here would be the way in which the courts have welcomed decision-making by ethics committees in hospitals as a preferable route to having these kinds of cases continuously adjudicated in the courts.

Would it be a compelling regulatory reason that we find differential treatment unacceptable and have to avoid it, if only by insisting on uniform process by convention? That might be true in a decentralized system, but it seems even more likely to be true in a national health care system. In Britain, for example, it might seem more troubling that Groucho did not get his transplant in London but Harpo got his in Manchester. Here too, however, there might be disagreements among *meaningful political units,* the districts, about what constituted the "best" decision-making procedure. If that is true, then there might be even more reason to tolerate variation than there is in the United States where people are grouped into insurance schemes, not meaningful political units that have ways of selecting their procedures in a democratic fashion.

How acceptable differential treatment would be seems to depend, then, on whether a persuasive political rationale for uniformity can be developed. In a decentralized system, the political rationale would have to be sufficient to override the presumption that private insurers or different states have the authority to select from among a set of comparably fair procedures. Of course, the political rationale might simply be that the legal system would not allow differential treatment. But that too remains to be seen.

In a national health care system, the political rationale for uniformity would have to show that differential treatment among districts was less acceptable than giving them the autonomy to select their own procedures. If meaningful political units, like districts, felt strongly enough about their choices of procedures, the costs of uniformity might be too high. For the problem we are facing, then, it remains unclear how unacceptable it would be for Harpo to get a last chance when Groucho does not.

LEARNING FROM THE EXPERIMENT

Making decisions and policies about payment for promising but unproven last-chance therapies presents the most difficult moral and clinical policy challenge a health care system can face. Important values, all of which command respect and attention, inevitably come into conflict in these difficult situations, especially giving some (how much?) priority to meeting the urgent claims of patients in last-chance situations, providing stewardship of collective resources, producing the public good of scientific knowledge about the effectiveness of unproven therapies, and respecting patient autonomy through collaborative decision-making about risks and benefits.

General principles of distributive justice do not tell us how to weigh the relative claims of these competing considerations. Nevertheless, the insurers and MCOs whose programs we describe have developed procedures for making decisions and policies that can be defended on the basis of justifiable, although different, weights they give to the different values. In our decentralized, competitive system—largely in response to political and legal pressures patients and clinicians have focused on these plans—an important social experiment has emerged. Different procedural solutions to the problem of limit setting in the case of new technologies are being developed and honed in practice. What can we learn from the experiment?

A harried health plan medical director in the United States or a district health officer in the British National Health Service might respond, "All your talk about accountability and giving different weights to different values doesn't help me at all! I have to make decisions in real time about real people with real life-threatening illnesses. If your work on setting limits fairly is worth anything, it should give me guidance about the right thing to do."

We take this complaint seriously. While our study of Aetna, Health Partners, Kaiser Permanente of Northern California, and Oregon Blue Cross Blue Shield does not suggest a single right policy for last-chance therapies, neither does it suggest a situation of extreme relativity, or "anything goes." All four programs gave significant—though differing—weight to urgent claims, stewardship, scientific knowledge, and patient autonomy. It is hard to imagine a justifiable policy approach that does not seriously engage with each of these values. Thus, while our reliance on fair process does not yield a single substantive conclusion for setting policy about last-chance therapies, it substantially narrows the range of acceptable possibilities. Our advice to the medical director or district health officer would be, "Go back to your key stakeholders, deliberate about how you want to balance the four key values, explain the reasons for your policy to the public, and start to apply it."

If we as a society can tolerate the inevitable differences in decisions and policies that various configurations of values will create, we will have an opportunity to learn from the dialectic between principles and practice. We will see more clearly, through a legacy of specific decisions and their outcomes, just what the moral and nonmoral benefits and costs of various approaches are. What we learn will help us refine our notions of fair procedure and in turn help us produce better solutions to the general problem of limit setting in health care that all societies are struggling with. In the last 20 to 30 years, we have learned much and seen important changes in how individual clinicians and patients negotiate the difficult issues of clinical planning in the context of threats to life itself. If we have enough societal fortitude, and a modicum of strong political leadership, close study of the experiences generated by the kinds of programs we have described can help us do the same at the level of social policy.

NOTES

1. It is important to distinguish the case of promising but unproven last-chance therapies, which are marked by uncertainty, from the case of treatments that professionals agree are futile.

2. The MAP criteria are cited in the previous chapter. The South African study (Bezwoda et al., 1995) used as its control a regimen of standard chemotherapy that was inferior in outcomes to the conventional therapy that was typically available in the United States and elsewhere. Showing that high-dose chemotherapy was superior to a regimen that itself was inferior to the conventional therapy commonly in use should not persuade us of the superior efficacy of the high dose regimen.

3. The California Blue Shield evaluation took place in a public setting, the only such open technology assessment process that we know of aside from Oregon Health Resources Commission. At its discussion, the panel seemed comfortable supporting its conclusion only after it was assured that no one actually wanting the high-dose chemotherapy was unable to get it, despite its investigational status.

6

LUNG VOLUME REDUCTION SURGERY: A CASE STUDY

As the previous chapters indicate, we developed our ideas about accountability for reasonableness out of a combination of field studies of health programs in action, philosophical analysis, and application of the concept in the course of doing a series of policy consultations in the United States and abroad. From 1995 to 1998 our field studies focused on how U.S. insurers and managed care organizations make policy about coverage of new technologies. We chose to investigate new technologies for three reasons. First, new technologies are a central component of both the promise and the cost of health care. As such, technology policy is an important focus of study in itself. Second, virtually all insurers and managed care organizations have committees and other explicit processes for making policy about the use of new technologies. This made it easier to study how policy is made—by observing committee meetings, reviewing minutes and other documents, and interviewing key participants.

Finally, decisions about new technologies involve the most rigorous and sophisticated efforts to decide policy on the basis of scientific evidence. Modern medical practice is founded on science, and the movement for evidence-based practice aims to have clinical and policy decisions made on empirical grounds. Thus, when we asked the scientific advisor to the new technology committee of a major insurer how our project could best contribute to the field, he said, "Identify the hurdle of evidence a new technology must pass to be covered." Many others whom we inter-viewed expressed the same wish for a "gold standard" of scientific evidence that insurers and managed care organizations could apply to determine whether or not they should cover a new technology.

This chapter argues that while it may be possible to create a gold standard for reaching conclusions about the *efficacy* of a new technology, the hope that the methods of evidence-based practice would tell us whether to *cover* that technol-ogy under insurance is quixotic. Evidence is crucial for making fair policy about new technologies, but it is not enough. Accountability for reasonableness emerges as a necessary component for setting fair and legitimate limits even in the domain of this most empirical methodology.

At the time of our field work on new technology policy, all of the programs we were working with were evaluating lung volume reduction surgery (LVRS), a new surgical procedure for emphysema, and deciding whether or not to cover it. Issues surrounding this surgery provide an unusually rich opportunity to investigate how insurers and managed care organizations decide about coverage. Because new sur-gical techniques do not require Food and Drug Administration (FDA) approval, insurers and managed care organizations have had to take full responsibility for coverage decisions about LVRS without prescreening by any official body. The fact that differently structured programs—for-profit and not-for-profit—in differ-ent parts of the country were all making policy about the same technology at the same time allowed us to examine the impact of program structure and local envi-ronment on decision-making.

Each of the programs at which we studied policy making for LVRS used a care-ful and thoughtful process. Although they made similar assessments of the empir-ical literature about LVRS, they reached different conclusions about coverage. None of the programs made their coverage decisions in an explicitly comparative context that considered trade-offs and opportunity costs. It was as if covering a new treatment carried no opportunity costs! We concluded that applying account-ability for reasonableness to policy making about LVRS could reduce the likeli-hood that carefully considered policies would be seen as capricious and arbitrary and would improve societal learning and the policy making process itself.

As with the last-chance cancer therapies discussed in Chapter 5, the evidence for the effectiveness of LVRS was strong but not definitive. There are, however, important differences between LVRS and last-chance therapies. LVRS lacks the "cure versus death" drama of last-chance technologies. LVRS is not believed to extend longevity, but it offers the potential for improved quality of life to patients with serious impairments. As such, it exemplifies a broad range of policy decisions in which it may be possible to achieve varying improvements in quality of life for a potentially significant increase of expenditure. Although last-chance technolo-gies attract more public attention and provide more frequent examples for ethics class discussions, the kinds of policy questions posed by LVRS will become ever more frequent as the global population ages and the science and technology under-lying medical practice progresses.

LUNG VOLUME REDUCTION SURGERY

Emphysema is a common lung disease that causes shortness of breath, progressive limitation of activity, and increased mortality. Cigarette smoking is the commonest cause. In emphysema the air spaces (alveoli) enlarge and the alveolar walls, through which respiration occurs, are destroyed. Chronic bronchitis—inflammation of the airway passages that lead to the alveoli—often occurs at the same time. An esti-mated 1.6 million Americans have emphysema, resulting in approximately 15,000 deaths a year. Emphysema increases in prevalence with age. The largest number of cases occurs in later mid-life and after 65.

Advanced emphysema causes severe suffering, especially shortness of breath, limited exercise capacity, and a nightmare-like feeling of suffocation or air hun-ger. Medical treatments for advanced emphysema provide limited benefit, and "frequently leave the patient in anguish and the physician frustrated" (Yusen & Lefrak, 1996, p. 83). Surgeons have tried to fill that gap in ways that have been aggressive, creative, and occasionally rash. Since the early 1900s, there has been a recurrent cycle of hope and disappointment in which one procedure after another has been tried, described initially as promising, but ultimately found to be inef-fective.

Lung volume reduction surgery is largely associated with the work of Dr. Joel Cooper, chief of cardiothoracic surgery at Washington University in St. Louis. Cooper's approach is far and away the best described and most extensively stud-ied surgical procedure for treating advanced emphysema.

Cooper—the leading advocate for LVRS—is fully aware of, and explicit about, the checkered history of surgical treatment of emphysema. In the first paragraph of an early article about LVRS (Cooper & Patterson, 1996), he refers to the numer-ous surgical approaches that have been tried:

> Each procedure was enthusiastically embraced for a time by its proponents, based on anecdotal reports of subjective improvement. However, the lack of consistent, objec-tively documented benefit caused each procedure to be discarded in turn.

By putting his own reports and advocacy into the context of precedents, Cooper does a small piece of education about the lessons of history, saying, in effect, "History shows us a cycle of hope, belief, and disappointment, so we must learn lessons from that history, apply them to the current situation, and demonstrate that we have done so." By identifying the key lessons of history and showing that specific efforts have been made to apply them to the development of LVRS, Cooper is able to argue forcefully that LVRS is not simply the latest example of surgical panacea for advanced emphysema.

The idea that reducing the size of the emphysematous lung might improve breathing was developed by Dr. Otto Brantigan at the University of Maryland in the late 1950s (Brantigan, Mueller, & Kress, 1959). Brantigan hypothesized that when a person with normal lungs breathes in, the elastic pull of the lung tissue widens the air passages (bronchi), but that in an expanded emphysematous lung, the elasticity diminishes and the airways tend to narrow or collapse when the patient breathes in. Brantigan reasoned that reducing lung volume by removing portions of the emphysematous lung would restore some of the lost elasticity, allowing the lungs to pull the narrowed airway passages open, and that reducing the volume of the lungs might allow the diaphragm to rise more vigorously. Both of these changes would improve respiration. Brantigan tried his procedure, but although it was promising, too many patients died during surgery and post-operatively for it to be used widely

In the intervening years, however, surgical, anesthetic, and postoperative care for patients with severe lung disease improved substantially, largely due to experience with lung transplantation, an area in which Cooper was a pioneer. The essential concept of LVRS is simple: the surgeon gains access to the chest cavity and then does something to reduce the volume of the enlarged emphysematous lungs. The multiple surgical techniques differ in *how* they gain access to the lungs and *what* technique(s) they use to reduce the volume of lung tissue.

Cooper and his colleagues at Barnes Hospital started their LVRS program in January 1993 and have accumulated patients at the rate of approximately one per week since then. A key feature of policy development for coverage of LVRS is that outcome results have emerged in a rolling fashion, with publication in peer-reviewed journals lagging behind public presentations by months to years.

Several of our collaborating sites reported that they began to consider covering LVRS after hearing Cooper present initial results at the April 1994 meeting of the American Association of Thoracic Surgery, nine months before he first published results in a peer-reviewed journal. That first publication, which appeared in January 1995, two years after the inception of the program, reported on 20 patients who had been followed for a mean of six months (Cooper, Trulock, Phol et al., 1996). One year later, in January 1996, the St. Louis group reported on 84 patients, 37 of whom had been followed for six months and 19 for one year (Yusen, Trulock, Phol et al., 1996). Three months later, in April 1996, in a debate about the status of LVRS (Cooper & Lefrak, 1996), Cooper summarized the first two-and-a-half years of the Barnes program, with findings from 120 patients followed for a mean of 375 days. All of the studies showed substantial and sustained improvement.

In the April 1996 debate, Cooper argued that LVRS should be made available to patients outside of research settings and should not be considered "investigational" for insurance coverage purposes. He asserted that waiting for publication in peer-reviewed publications was an inappropriate standard to apply because of the inevitable delays that peer review entails. Cooper acknowledged that LVRS had not been subjected to randomized trials, but argued that, because patients who received intensive pulmonary rehabilitation and optimal medical therapy while awaiting transplantation reached a plateau after approximately two months, a randomized trial comparing ongoing medical treatment and pulmonary rehabilitation to LVRS was not required to establish the surgery's efficacy.

Taking the negative position, Make and Albert (1996) agreed that LVRS was "promising." They argued, however, that LVRS should be held to the standard of whether the available evidence allowed physicians and patients to "carefully and rationally choose the most appropriate tests and procedures based on a careful assessment of the demonstrated risks, benefits, and costs." In their view, LVRS had not yet met this standard. On that basis Make and Albert concluded that "[the] prudent course is to await further information prior to recommending this treatment to our patients."

In an excellent analysis entitled "Lessons from Lung Volume Reduction Surgery," Tonelli (Tonelli, Benditt, & Albert, 1996) argued that the evidence for the efficacy of LVRS (as of mid-1996) was at a point of "clinical equipoise" (Freedman, 1987). In equipoise, equally well-informed experts could reasonably disagree as to whether Cooper was right in asserting that the procedure had been evaluated enough to be presented to patients as an established treatment alternative or whether Make and Albert were correct that it should still be seen as investigational. In other words, the situation for LVRS in 1996 was analogous to what is often seen in the courtroom, when dueling experts present conflicting scientific testimony to a perplexed jury. Individual experts of high integrity and equivalent scientific credentials may have been passionately committed to their views of the scientific status of LVRS, but unless they could agree on a single gold standard for coverage, conflict between them would be essentially unresolvable by debate about the evidence.

"To Cover or Not to Cover—That Is the Question"

The scientific and clinical findings about a new technology or treatment are disseminated ever more rapidly to a national and even international audience through professional meetings, media reports of those meetings, peer-reviewed journals, and, increasingly, the Internet. In the mixed U.S. health care system, these findings are processed and acted on by a mixture of local/regional/national insurance and managed care programs, public and private, and not-for-profit and for-profit. All programs have access to the same scientific and clinical data, but they operate under a diversity of internal structures and external market conditions.

Not surprisingly, we found a comparably diverse policy response among the programs we studied. Two—Health Partners and PacifiCare—chose not to cover

LVRS other than by exception on a case-by-case basis. Five—Aetna, Blue Cross Blue Shield of Oregon, Group Health Cooperative of Puget Sound, Harvard Pilgrim Health Care, and Northern California Kaiser Permanente—developed policies that essentially "approve" or "adopt" LVRS under guidelines that determine where, when, and for whom the procedure should be used. The most national program of all—Medicare—did something altogether different.

The contrast between Health Partners in Minnesota and Northern California Kaiser Permanente is especially interesting. Both organizations are highly respected, not-for-profit HMOs, with strong traditions of evidence-based practice. Given the state of "clinical equipoise," it was not startling that these two outstanding organizations would make different policy decisions for LVRS. But the fact that acting on the same evidence and very similar analyses of the evidence, they arrived at different conclusions at what was essentially the same time provides an excellent opportunity to study the determinants of what Wennberg (1988) calls "local area variation" at the level of coverage policy.

Although Washington University is the site of the most extensive ongoing scientific study of LVRS, California—especially Southern California—rapidly became the Lourdes-like pilgrimage site for LVRS. One journalist described Orange County as "something of a Mecca for desperate emphysema patients hoping to breathe again with ease," (Greene, 1996) and another spoke of "lung surgeries that draw hundreds of desperate emphysema sufferers each year" (Marquis, 1996). A pulmonologist in Seattle reported receiving a direct mail solicitation from one of the California centers claiming that "excellent functional results with acceptable perioperative morbidity and mortality have been demonstrated with this procedure" (quoted in Tonelli et al., 1996)—a claim that went far beyond what any of the academic clinical and research leaders were saying at the time.

Given the entrepreneurial environment that was giving LVRS such a hard sell in California, it is not surprising that the minutes of an October 26, 1995, Northern California Kaiser Permanente meeting to consider LVRS note that "[t]here are increasing numbers of centers in the [Northern California Region] service area where volume reduction surgery is provided." In an interview, a senior staff member commented that, in northern California, "people just won't wait until the end of the Health Care Financing Agency (HCFA) study [see below] . . . if Kaiser tried not to cover LVRS it wouldn't last 10 seconds in the court of public opinion." The leadership at Kaiser perceived very strong patient demand and provider push for LVRS in the organization's service area.

In addition to strong external demand, Northern California Kaiser Permanente had strong internal champions within the medical group, including a thoracic surgeon who had done five LVRS procedures as of late 1995 and who was part of the medical group management structure. The agenda for the October meeting reflected the positive internal attitude towards LVRS and presupposed that the procedure had moved beyond the investigational phase: "The purpose of this meeting is to share information about experiences with volume reduction surgery and patient outcomes, to develop consensus among [Permanente Medical Group] physicians regarding the medical appropriateness of these procedures for individually selected patients, and to agree on site(s) for provision of these services." This was a meeting to determine *how* to offer LVRS, not *whether* to offer it.

The group convened to consider LVRS was defined as "an interdisciplinary clinical expert group," consisting of two pulmonologists, five thoracic surgeons, one intensivist, and three generalist-managers. The group identified as its "greatest concern the potential for overutilization of the surgery in outside centers operating on patients in whom the procedure is not medically appropriate." It elected to follow a "Center of Excellence" strategy and recommended providing LVRS at a single site within the Northern California Kaiser Permanente program that could ensure the crucial surgical, anesthetic, pulmonological, nursing and rehabilitative expertise and could collect data in an rigorous manner.

Northern California Kaiser Permanente is the oldest prepaid group practice in the United States, with longer experience providing care within defined resource limits than even the British National Health Service (NHS). It was therefore establishing its policy for LVRS within a very cohesive and, by U.S. standards, extremely well-managed group practice. It could approach the situation of clinical equipoise regarding evidence, uncertain clinical indications, and rapid technical change, with confidence that the provision of LVRS would be under the wing of well-informed specialists who were committed to the norms of the capitated group practice. The leadership did not fear that provision of LVRS would get out of control, as they believed it had elsewhere in the state.

In mid-February 1996, four months after Northern California Kaiser Permanente decided to provide LVRS for carefully selected patients within its own care system, the medical directors' committee at Health Partners of Minnesota decided not to cover the procedure. If anything, the fact of making the coverage decision in February 1996, as opposed to October 1995, could have tilted the process towards a positive coverage decision, since the Washington University group had published a series of five papers, including an updated outcome study, in the January 1996 issue of *Seminars in Thoracic and Cardiovascular Surgery* (Cooper & Patterson, 1996).

On September 29, 1995, the Institute for Clinical Systems Integration (ICSI), an independent technology assessment and guideline development organization associated with Health Partners, issued a report on LVRS. Like the expert group that made LVRS policy for Northern California Kaiser Permanente, the ICSI work group consisted of pulmonologists and thoracic surgeons. The report classified the evidence for LVRS as a case series (the lowest level of evidence ICSI recognizes), and concluded that "longer-term data are critical before assessment of safety and efficacy of [LVRS] is possible." The body of the report, however, characterized LVRS in terms as positive as those used in the Northern California Kaiser Permanente decision-making process: [T]he results to date . . . show a *definite* improvement in lung function, exercise tolerance and psychosocial status. . . . [T]he short term results of bilateral (volume reduction) pneumectomy surgery appear *promising*. . . . [P]atients *requiring* lung reduction surgery should be enrolled in carefully designed scientifically valid clinical trials. [emphasis added] (Institute for Clinical Systems Integration, 1995).

Findings of this kind could certainly have provided Health Partners with a rationale for covering LVRS for selected patients at selected centers of excellence conducting scientific trials as Northern California Kaiser Permanente had decided to do. Health Partners and Northern California Kaiser Permanente reviewed the same evidence and assessed it as consisting of a case series. Both organizations identified uncertainty about the long-term effectiveness of LVRS as a major concern. Both identified the absence of clear criteria to predict which patients will benefit as a problem.

In other words, Health Partners and Northern California Kaiser Permanente did not make different policy for LVRS on the basis of access to different evidence or different assessments of the evidence itself. The fact that they made similar assessments of the efficacy of the new treatment was consistent with the hope that there might be a gold standard of evidence that could determine whether or not to cover a new technology. The key factors in their making opposite decisions about coverage appear to be differences in the California and Minnesota environments, different weight being given to different values, and subtle differences in the policy-making process at the two organizations.

With regard to the local environment, the Minnesota public displayed significantly less demand for LVRS than did the public in California. Although the University of Minnesota and the Mayo Clinic were both doing LVRS in 1995, there was essentially no entrepreneurial marketing of the procedure in Minnesota as there was in California. Prior to HCFA's setting a national non-coverage policy for LVRS in December 1995 [see below], Minnesota had been the only state that had explicitly not covered LVRS under Medicare, so the over-65 population had not had much experience with the procedure and did not expect it to be covered. Finally, in terms of values, Minneapolis has an unusually strong and well-organized business community purchaser group that had, in effect, asked Minnesota insurers to apply high standards of evidence in making coverage policy. Even though northern California is historically an older managed-care market, Minneapolis appears to have more of an evidence-based, tight management ethos. In a state of clinical equipoise regarding evidence, the Minnesota environment favored a conservative approach.

With regard to the policy making process, Health Partners pursues a strict separation of technology assessment and policy making about the adoption and application of a new technology. Different groups do the technology assessment and the making of coverage policy, and the technology assessment is actually done at a separate organization (ICSI). Like Northern California Kaiser Permanente, the technology assessment was done by pulmonologists and thoracic surgeons, supported by specialized technology assessment staff. However, compared to Northern California Kaiser Permanente, pulmonologists and thoracic surgeons played a less direct role in setting the coverage policy at Health Partners. While specialists were in the majority at the Northern California Kaiser Permanente meeting at which policy was set, the policy-setting meeting at Health Partners included only generalist physicians with management responsibilities. Although the policy-making group had solicited comments from specialists, no specialists were actually present, and the minutes do not suggest that specialist comments played a major role in the deliberations.

Between the majority presence of thoracic surgeons and pulmonologists in the group that made policy for LVRS at Northern California Kaiser Permanente, and the fact that the policy was for an integrated group practice (self-management), the California coverage policy decision-making process appears to have been conducted in accord with the maxim: Although the evidence for LVRS is in a state of clinical equipoise, the patient indications are unclear, and the long-term impact has not been established, the procedure is very promising. Since we can count on our group to apply LVRS with great care, carefully track what happens, stay within the boundaries of what is known, and modify the program in accord with our findings and research done elsewhere, let's cover it.

Between the absence of thoracic surgeons and pulmonologists in the group that made policy for LVRS at Health Partners and the fact that the policy was for independent physicians and groups (management of others) as well as its own integrated group practice, the Minnesota policy making appears to have been conducted in accord with the maxim: The evidence for LVRS is in a state of clinical equipoise, the patient indications are unclear, and the long term impact has not been established. Even though LVRS is a promising technology, let's be sure to recognize the embryonic state of what is known, hold to a policy of non-coverage for the present, and wait to see how the research evolves.

Northern California Kaiser Permanente emphasized the promising side of the evidence in its policy, and Health Partners emphasized the uncertainties. The different conclusions they reached did not arise from different technology assessments or different understandings of evidence based practice. Rather, it appears that differences in the *1)* level of member demand; *2)* presence or absence of strong internal champions for the procedure; *3)* practice patterns and beliefs in Minnesota and California; *4)* intensity of the role of specialists who might advocate for the procedure in the policy-making process; *5)* degree to which the organization making policy felt confident of its capacity to manage the policy-implementation process; and, *6)* as discussed in greater detail in the chapter on last-chance technologies, the relative weight given to different values, all contributed substantially to the different policy outcomes for the two HMOs.

Based on these differences in local environment and guiding values, Northern California Kaiser Permanente and Health Partners applied different standards to the evidence for determining whether the evidence was good enough to justify coverage. Within its own framework and circumstances, each HMO could justify the claim that it made the right answer. The Northern California Kaiser Permanente/Health Partners story indicates that even if the clinical community adopts a gold standard for assessing clinical and research evidence for *efficacy,* there is no gold standard for determining *coverage* in the context of a complex, multifactorial decision-making process.

In public discussion of health care policy, one often encounters the assumption that for-profit insurers will be monolithically driven by concern about the bottom line. Our field study suggests that reality is much more complex than this stereotype would suggest, since the two for-profit organizations we worked with—Aetna and PacifiCare—differed in their coverage policy for LVRS.

Aetna put a positive coverage policy in place on March 22, 1996. Its policy statement described the Barnes Hospital program in detail and adopted the selection criteria, preoperative work-up and surgical approach used at Barnes. It limited coverage to institutions with the same level of anesthesia, nursing, surgical, and pulmonology skills as Barnes. At several site visits, nurses responsible for liaison with insurers told us that getting coverage for LVRS through Aetna was essentially "hassle free" when the patient's condition met the clinical criteria. In other words, Aetna coverage policy appeared to be filtering down to the front line.

PacifiCare, in contrast, concluded on November 16, 1995, that LVRS lacked "conclusive evidence from well-controlled trials [that showed] improvement in health outcomes" and that "no studies comparing LVRS and pulmonary rehabilitation have been reported." Because the corporate headquarters are located in Orange County, the leadership of PacifiCare was keenly aware of anecdotes about terrible outcomes from locally prescribed LVRS. These incidents, combined with an assessment of the evidence similar to the one made by the leadership at Health Partners, led PacifiCare to promulgate a policy under which LVRS was not a covered benefit. PacifiCare continues to review requests for LVRS on a case-by-case basis and is prepared to make an exception if persuaded by specific clinical circumstances, but its global policy remains one of non-coverage.

A single case study does not allow broad conclusions about the impact of for-profit status on health care policy. But the fact that Kaiser Permanente of Northern California (not-for-profit) and Aetna (for-profit) both chose to cover LVRS, while Health Partners (not-for-profit) and PacifiCare (for-profit) did not, shows that, at least for LVRS, for-profit status does not determine coverage policy.

The scientific advisor to a new technology committee who asked us to "identify the hurdle of evidence a new technology must pass to be covered" and the others who expressed the wish for a "gold standard" of evidence were articulating the dream that coverage policy could be derived from evidence. As necessary as evi-

dence is for coverage decisions, our study of LVRS indicates that it is not sufficient. The policy controversy about LVRS coverage was not about what the evidence was, but what its implications for policy should be. This is essentially the
familiar distinction between "is" and "ought." When a low-cost intervention provides tremendous benefit or a high-cost intervention provides microscopically tiny
benefits, it is easy to confuse the "is" of evidence with the "ought" of policy. If
an asteroid were about to crash into the earth, and the most promising asteroid-
busting technique was supported by evidence a fraction as good as the evidence
for LVRS, the asteroid-buster would immediately be "covered" for deployment.
While there can be a gold standard for reaching conclusions about efficacy, the nature of the question the evidence is being used to help decide, and the values at
play in the decision-making environment, determine the height of the evidence
hurdle required for coverage. In a health system with as much diversity as is found
in the United States, a gold standard for moving from evidence ("is") to coverage
("ought") is a pipe dream. As central as it is, evidence does not obviate the need
for a fair process.

GUARDIAN OF THE PUBLIC TRUST: HCFA MAKES LVRS
POLICY FOR THE MEDICARE POPULATION

Every insurer has a moral as well as contractual responsibility for its insured population, but among insurers, the HCFA is special. HCFA represents our societal
commitment to the elderly and disabled, the groups with greatest health needs in
the general population. Except for the relatively small number of disabled whose
disabilities abate, Medicare is a commitment for life. It is the sole insurance program through which the United States guarantees health care to its citizens.

Because emphysema is more common among the elderly, coverage for LVRS is
inevitably a crucial policy question for Medicare. The issue of LVRS first got onto
the HCFA agenda in May 1995, when, at a meeting of the HCFA Technology
Advisory Committee (TAC), one of the state Medicare carrier medical directors
reported receiving claims for a procedure called "lung shaving" and asked what
others knew about it.

Except for the carrier medical director from St. Louis, who was familiar with
the LVRS program at Barnes Hospital, few present at the TAC meeting had
much knowledge about LVRS. A HCFA staff member was asked to do research
on LVRS and reported at the July 1995 TAC meeting that only one published
reference—Cooper's January 1995 paper that described his initial experience with
20 patients—was in the peer-reviewed literature. At the same meeting, a number
of those present reported anecdotes of bad outcomes when LVRS was done at hospitals without the necessary levels of anesthetic, surgical, and postoperative care.

Without being aware of what was happening, Medicare had actually been covering LVRS. Bills were being submitted under established procedure codes, including "wedge resection" and "bullectomy," which were approved procedures for other indications. Once it became clear that LVRS was being done relatively widely, and that, without having established a policy about LVRS, Medicare had unwittingly been paying for it, HCFA determined that it needed an explicit policy.

An observer of the HCFA process from May through December 1995 commented that "HCFA couldn't really go out with a policy of general coverage for LVRS on the basis of one article by Dr. Cooper at a time that anecdotes were coming in about bad outcomes elsewhere," given that "HCFA's patients with emphysema are a very special population, different than what the insurance companies see. . . . They are older and have multiple comorbidities. . . . On average, HCFA's patients are sicker and more vulnerable."

From HCFA's national perspective, promising work at Barnes Hospital with a somewhat younger population and a rigorous program of preoperative evaluation, postsurgical follow-up and data collection well beyond what any other centers were doing, did not allow for a responsible "yes" answer to the question of whether Medicare would cover LVRS for the thousands of patients who would surely seek the treatment at the scores or hundreds of centers that would offer it. Consequently, in December 1995, HCFA issued an initial "instruction" that LVRS for emphysema would not be covered as of January 1, 1996.

However, the initial "no" answer to the question of LVRS coverage was also not seen within HCFA as an adequate policy response. While HCFA did not regard LVRS as ready for unrestricted coverage, the procedure appeared to be a promising technology for a condition of great importance to the Medicare population. A senior HCFA official commented, "To put it bluntly, if one was to subject most services, new or old, to the criteria of evidence-based medicine, the evidence for just about every service would be found deficient. As the nation's largest payer we can't have an evidence-based process that would require us to simply give yes or no answers."

To address this dilemma, HCFA has created a "coverage with conditions" category of response. HCFA cannot meet its responsibilities to the Medicare population if it is limited to the blunt instrument of either saying "Yes, we will cover this technology," or "No, we will not cover it." "Coverage with conditions" allows HCFA to specify patient and facility selection criteria and to require other parameters of the sort that go into treatment guidelines. The same official commented that "if we waited for definitive data, we wouldn't do anything," but "if we cover a technology too early, it becomes so widespread that you can't compare it to anything else and know how well it works." The "coverage with conditions" response is an effort to "put in a little wedge between the investigational phase and the application phase."

One way of implementing a "coverage with conditions" policy would be through a "Center of Excellence" approach, under which LVRS would be covered at designated sites, characterized by appropriate expertise and commitment to conducting scientifically acceptable systematic evaluations. HCFA had followed this strategy with heart and lung transplantation, but these are procedures limited by the availability of organs, and therefore not susceptible to the same wide dissemination as LVRS. According to a HCFA spokesperson, for a public program like HCFA to restrict the eligible sites for delivery of LVRS as required by a Center of Excellence strategy, "We would have to develop criteria, collect data, and have public comment in the Federal Register. While we have an exceptionally qualified staff, this would take an enormous effort to do."

The experience of Oregon Blue Cross Blue Shield, which did chose to cover LVRS for its non-Medicare insurees under a Center of Excellence approach, suggests that even if HCFA had wished to pursue a similar strategy, it is highly unlikely it could have done so successfully. Oregon is a small service delivery area, with a limited number of hospitals that might compete to provide LVRS and, as of 1996, when the positive coverage policy was set, had no entrepreneurial lung center development of the sort seen in California.

Despite the relative simplicity of the environment in Oregon, implementing a Center of Excellence coverage strategy for LVRS was difficult. The first step was to change the name from "Center of Excellence" to "participating center" in order to eliminate the potential implication that a non-participant is not "excellent." The Oregon Blue Cross Blue Shield medical director traveled across the state, meeting with pulmonologists and thoracic surgeons to cultivate support for a policy of participating centers. It was a labor-intensive, consensus-building, political process. Success depended on personal trust and understanding the local ecology of health services. HCFA insures a fortyfold larger population than Oregon Blue Cross Blue Shield and, as a public entity, is subjected to intense political pressures and lobbying efforts. A Center of Excellence strategy is simply not a strategy that HCFA could realistically implement.

Concomitant with issuance of its initial non-coverage policy in January 1996, HCFA requested a formal assessment of the safety and efficacy of LVRS from the Center for Health Care Technology (CHCT) at the federal Agency for Health Care Policy and Research. CHCT collected information from 26 sites that responded to the request for information. These sites together had accumulated 3,000 cases of LVRS, but only Barnes Hospital had systematically followed all of the patients undergoing the procedure. CHCT commented on the "vanishing denominators" in the studies and concluded that the accuracy of the data was unreliable when large numbers of patients were lost to follow-up. The study "found the data inconclusive regarding the risks and benefits of [LVRS], and recommended limited Medicare reimbursement as part of a national study of the procedure" (*HHS News,* 1996).

On the basis of this recommendation, HCFA implemented an innovative policy for LVRS. In the face of explosive development of entrepreneurial lung centers and rapid dissemination of LVRS well beyond centers able to deliver it in a medically responsible manner, a policy of coverage would have allowed unacceptably poor patient care, stifled further scientific study of LVRS, and wasted public money. A policy of total non-coverage would have overlooked the promising dimensions of LVRS that had led a majority of our collaborating sites to positive coverage decisions, and which led the Blue Cross Blue Shield Association's National Technology Evaluation Center to conclude[1] that LVRS met its evaluation criteria when done at institutions with appropriate levels of skill under Cooper's patient selection criteria (Technology Evaluation Center, 1996). Insurers like Oregon Blue Cross Blue Shield and Aetna and managed care organizations like Northern California Kaiser Permanente were politically able to bridge the dilemma of "yes" versus "no" policy responses with carefully managed forms of a Center of Excellence strategy. By our analysis, however, HCFA could not do the same for a technology like LVRS that does not have an absolute ceiling on its use imposed by limited organ availability.

In this context, HCFA joined with the National Heart, Lung, and Blood Institute (NHLBI) to sponsor a seven-year randomized controlled trial that will compare LVRS plus optimal medical therapy to optimal medical therapy alone. Patients will be enrolled at selected clinical centers with Johns Hopkins University serving as the coordinating center for the study. The data will be reviewed regularly, so if trends emerge before the planned end of the study, coverage policy can be adjusted. If LVRS proves to be more effective than skeptics believe, in seven years, family members who have lost a relative whose quality of life and possibly even longevity might have been extended will be bitter. If LVRS proves to be more variable in its outcomes and more dangerous to patients than its advocates believe, patients and families who might have undergone the procedure and suffered currently unknown harms will be grateful. As described in Chapter 5, ABMT for advanced breast cancer was widely disseminated before an adequate evaluation had been done, and when the facts emerged it turned out to be no better—and possibly worse—than standard therapy. HCFA was determined not to repeat that situation with LVRS.

Given the fact that the insurers and managed care organizations who collaborated with us came to different conclusions regarding coverage for LVRS despite having access to the same published data base, it was not surprising that the initial meetings of the steering committee for the HCFA-financed NHLBI study evinced the same conflicting views. Some participants, supported by the conclusion of the prestigious Blue Cross Blue Shield Technology Evaluation Center, had concluded that the efficacy of LVRS had been well enough established that a randomized controlled trial would be unethical. On the basis of this perspective, the Institutional Review Board at Barnes Hospital—where LVRS had been developed and most extensively studied—ultimately refused to approve participation in the study. Others believed that, while LVRS was promising, the long term results, clinical indications, and appropriate evaluation were at a level of uncertainty for which a randomized controlled trial was the proper scientific and policy response.

At a time when managing the future growth of Medicare expenditures is a central part of the effort to balance the federal budget, it would seem highly appropriate for the opportunity cost of providing LVRS under Medicare to be part of a public deliberation on HCFA's coverage policy. One estimate places the incremental cost of covering LVRS at approximately $5 billion (Albert, Lewis, Wood, et al., 1996). Costs of this magnitude have obvious relevance to the possibility of adding other new benefits, such as prescription coverage. At the time LVRS coverage was being discussed, however, explicit discussion of opportunity costs, trade-offs and possible rationing were essentially forbidden topics. The next section expands further on the issue of budgeting and tradeoffs.

"COMPARED TO WHAT?" THE ISSUE OF OPPORTUNITY COSTS

We began our field study of technology policy expecting to find insurers and managed care organizations considering opportunity costs and alternative uses of funds as a factor in their decisions about the adoption and application of new technologies. To our surprise, none of the seven collaborating sites at which we studied policy development for LVRS showed signs of any explicit consideration of true opportunity costs.

Interestingly, the clearest statement of the importance of considering opportunity costs in making policy about LVRS came from Cooper, the leading advocate for the procedure. In the debate, "Is volume reduction surgery appropriate in the treatment of emphysema?" after arguing vigorously for the "yes" position, Cooper added, "This does not mean that a cost-benefit assessment of the procedure is not required or that society would be willing to absorb the cost of expensive procedures that benefit a limited number of patients" (Cooper & Lefrak, 1996, p. 1203).

At one of the sites we studied (Harvard Pilgrim Health Care), the group responsible for making policy about the use of new technologies explicitly asked the expert panel reviewing the safety and efficacy of LVRS to assess the value of the benefit provided by LVRS relative to the cost. The expert panel, consisting of pulmonologists, a thoracic surgeon, and technology assessment experts, heard the question but did not address it at all, except that the surgeon did compare the cost of LVRS to the costs of treating *1)* chronic lung disease that no longer responded to medical treatment, *2)* lung transplant, and *3)* poorly done LVRS, which might be followed by a long intensive care unit (ICU) stay.

At a second site (Group Health Cooperative of Puget Sound), the pulmonologist who chaired the technology assessment group also compared the cost of LVRS to transplant, commenting that LVRS could be a significantly less costly alternative to transplant, but he made no comparisons of cost or value within or beyond the contrast between the two forms of surgery.

At a third site (Northern California Kaiser Permanente), the expert panel appears to have begun its deliberations already convinced that LVRS was a promising treatment that should be offered to patients with advanced emphysema who met appropriate eligibility criteria. That panel considered costs only from the perspective of the relative merits (quality and cost) of doing the procedure within the organization or on the outside (the "make or buy" question), and concluded that, in the entrepreneurial environment in which they were located, provision of LVRS by outside groups posed a danger of excessive utilization and provision of the procedure to patients for whom they believed the surgery was not indicated.

Given that emphysema, as a largely smoking-induced disorder, is in principle a preventable condition (Petty & Weinmann, 1997), it was surprising that the policy discussions of LVRS coverage did not include discussion of the choice between prevention and reparative strategies, especially given government and insurer efforts to recover health care costs from the tobacco industry through litigation. Since all of the organizations we studied make major investments in smoking prevention, to have included some reference to the choice between prevention and repair in the policy discussions might have been a useful further piece of public and provider education about opportunity costs in allocation of health care funds.

Our observations suggest that the expert panels that most of the organizations used to assess the safety and efficacy of LVRS, and which some used for making policy about adoption and application of LVRS, were not well suited for considering opportunity costs. The panels did make a small number of comparisons within the domain of pulmonology and thoracic surgery—to unresponsive pulmonary disease, transplant, poorly conducted LVRS, and clinically inappropriate, entrepreneurial provision of LVRS. However, even when explicitly asked to do so, none of the expert panels commented on the relative value of LVRS compared to any alternative use of funds, including using the funds for smoking prevention and cessation programs.

The example of Health Partners and ICSI suggests that decision-making groups composed of generalists may function significantly differently from groups composed of specialists. The specialty group that ICSI constituted to do a formal technology assessment of lung volume surgery assessed LVRS in much the same way that the organizations that ended up covering LVRS did. The enthusiastic tone of the report suggests that, if the specialist group at ICSI had been responsible for making policy about coverage, LVRS might have been covered, as it was at Northern California Kaiser Permanente.

To consider opportunity costs, a decision-making body must have a broad purview on the range of treatments the managed care organization provides and some kind of framework for making comparisons. Expert panels composed of specialists are not likely to have this kind of broad vision. The likeliest group to consider opportunity costs and trade-offs would be a decision-making group composed of generalists and other managers with a broad perspective on the entire range of organizational expenditures. While the generalist policy-making committee within Health Partners did not explicitly consider opportunity costs when it decided not to cover LVRS, the fact that it did not follow the potentially positive coverage implications of the ICSI report suggests that it had more capacity to take the kind of broad purview necessary for considering opportunity costs than the specialist group at ICSI did.

Cynics, critics, and much of the American public believe that managed care is excessively oriented to the bottom line and neglects patient welfare. A reviewer for one of the foundations that considered our project advised the foundation, "This is a worthless project. . . . There is nothing to study. . . . We all know that the only factor in making policy about new technologies is cost!" The fact that we did not observe explicit consideration of opportunity costs entering the decision-making process about whether to cover LVRS does not prove that cost was not a factor in making policy. However, the moral of this aspect of the LVRS story is that coverage policy is being made without explicit reference to competing priorities or alternative uses of funds outside of the domain of emphysema treatment.

As a result, the intelligent, careful, and labor-intensive work that our collaborators devoted to decision-making about coverage for LVRS did nothing to advance the health care system or society on a learning curve of increased capacity for handling trade-offs, making hard choices, or considering rationing. When we challenged them about the absence of consideration of opportunity costs, the sites uniformly responded that society has not given them sanction for making trade-offs. Rationing was an altogether forbidden topic. If we want insurers and managed care organizations to contribute to a societal learning curve, our political process will have to make the setting of limits an explicitly discussible subject. We cannot realistically expect insurers to take the lead in territory that political leaders have so scrupulously avoided entering.

CONCLUSION

Our key conclusion from this study of lung volume reduction surgery is that in a decentralized, pluralistic health care system, what counts as adequate evidence of treatment efficacy will vary with factors like local demand, clinician expectations, and degree of potential benefit for patients as well as the factor of giving different weights to different values that we emphasized in the discussion of last chance therapies. The study suggests that the scientific community can indeed come close to establishing a gold standard for evaluating the *efficacy* of a new treatment or technology. That evidence, and the gold standard used in assessing it, however, are only two of many considerations in making policy for *coverage*. As important as the quality of evidence is, it does not automatically trump all other considerations.

This conclusion will disappoint the harried health plan medical director and district health officer we invoked at the end of Chapter 5. For them, the commonsense view—Do what works and don't do what doesn't work—has great appeal. They might confront us with a new complaint: "You just make things worse and worse for us. If we can't rely on evidence to determine our decisions, we're lost!"

Once again our response would be that while accountability for reasonableness does not yield a single right answer to the question of whether or not to cover LVRS, it narrows the range of potential responses and suggests some practical approaches. All programs gave significant weight to the urgent claims of patients suffering with emphysema, stewardship, scientific knowledge and patient autonomy. Because LVRS was believed to affect (possibly) quality of life but to have no effect on longevity, all programs included the principle of "do no harm" as a prominent piece of their deliberations. Because of the potential for harm, all programs that elected to cover LVRS implemented some form of a Center of Excellence strategy. And, as a unique practical approach, HCFA expressed its commitment to developing better scientific knowledge about LVRS by covering it, but only in the context of a randomized trial.

As of the late 1990s, we found a striking lack of explicit comparison of the value of LVRS compared to other potential uses of the funds. Even in capitated programs, it were as if LVRS were being evaluated on its own merits, without consideration of opportunity costs or implications for trade-offs. We saw little evidence that insurers and managed care organizations were prepared to take the lead in moving society on a learning curve concerning dealing with health care limits. Their clear, consistent and plausible view was that this leadership must come from the political sphere.

An obvious objection to the conclusions we draw in this chapter is that they are based on a single case study. Our conclusions are not based on a survey or statistical analysis of coverage practices, but they are supported by two other case studies as well—the study of decision-making about autologous bone marrow transplant for advanced breast cancer that forms the basis of Chapter 5—and a study of decision-making about pallidotomy, a surgical procedure aimed at relieving the symptoms of advanced Parkinson's disease.[2]

In the case of pallidotomy, we found the following parallels to the LVRS case: *1)* there was a similar variation in coverage policy, in part driven by local variation in demand and in part by different weighing of the relevant values; *2)* there was again no consideration of opportunity costs, and costs were only considered through the development of "mini-guidelines" for when the procedure should be used; *3)* there was no single hurdle (gold standard) that, if cleared, made evidence "good enough" to require coverage; and, *4)* programs that covered the procedure did not simply say "Yes, we will cover it," but promulgated guidelines about patient selection and selection of provider sites.

Even if HCFA and the insurers and managed care organizations that we studied are not prepared to take political leadership off the hot seat by taking the lead in educating the public about the need for health care limits, they could still do significantly more to assume accountability for explaining the reasons for their policies. Each of the seven programs we studied conducted a policy-making process that focused on benefit for individual patients and the covered population. None had anything to be ashamed of or to want to hide. But a skeptical public, seeing that five covered LVRS and two did not, and that HCFA followed an altogether different path, largely concluded the worst—that policy-making was capricious and arbitrary or that money was the only concern. [Readers can sample the public skepticism and anger by exploring the Society for Thoracic Surgery discussion site for LVRS on the Web at http://www.sts.org/discuss/topics/discuss-lvrs.html.]

HCFA provides an especially clear example of how accountability for reasonableness could improve public understanding and the policy-making process. We believe that, in principle, Medicare could have decided to cover LVRS at Centers of Excellence under strict guidelines the way Aetna, Northern California Kaiser Permanente, and the other three programs did, but that political constraints made it impossible to implement such a policy choice. We concluded that, in its actual environment, the policy Medicare chose—a randomized controlled trial cosponsored with the National Heart, Lung, and Blood Institute—was a very reasonable course for HCFA to take.

Under accountability for reasonableness, if our analysis is correct, HCFA would have openly explained the rationale for its policy choice in this manner. Had they done so, critics of the HCFA policy could have targeted their advocacy more effectively. Instead of attacking HCFA for uncaring, callous policies, the critics could have focused on addressing the impediments to HCFA choosing a Center of Excellence strategy with strict guidelines and careful ongoing clinical study. Responding to the criticisms brought forward by the advocates, in July 2000, Senators William Frist, Edward Kennedy, and Arlen Specter asked HCFA to change its policy. If those senators understood the reasons why HCFA did not choose the Center of Excellence strategy in the first place they could have put their influence to work in dealing with the impediments. Without accountability for reasonableness, policy debate is much less able to engage with the real issues underlying policy choices. Participants in that debate—like the three senators—are less likely to focus their advocacy on the real problems, and society will not progress in learning how to deal with limits in a fair manner.

NOTES

1. In a remarkable coincidence, Blue Cross Blue Shield issued its policy at almost the exact time that CHCT concluded the data were "inconclusive" and recommended a randomized controlled trial!

2. We are indebted to Susann Wilkinson, who took the lead in our study of pallidotomy.

7

MAKING PHARMACY BENEFITS
ACCOUNTABLE FOR REASONABLENESS

Managing access to pharmaceuticals is a microcosm of the limit-setting problems in health care systems as a whole. Since most medical treatment includes the administration of pharmaceuticals, meeting needs for drugs fairly under resource constraints models the larger problem. If we are right that accountability for reasonableness is a solution to the legitimacy problem in health systems as a whole, then it should be possible to illustrate what such accountability would mean in practical terms in pharmacy benefit management. We address that challenge in this chapter.[1]

The challenge arises in any national health program or insurance system that provides a pharmacy benefit. In publicly administered systems abroad, pharmacy committees often construct a formulary, and coverage is provided for drugs in it. In some programs, criteria for inclusion are explicit, and criteria for how to use cost-effectiveness analyses may also be explicit. In general, however, the grounds for specific decisions are not routinely made public, violating the publicity requirement of accountability for reasonableness. Because the criteria for inclusion are not public, it is not clear whether the relevance requirement is satisfied, even if the criteria that were used had counted as relevant reasons. In any case, deliberation about the weights given to such reasons is not in general publicly accessible. The availability of adequate appeals procedures varies extensively by country. In our view, the challenge to make pharmacy benefits accountable for reasonableness in many publicly administered systems has only partially been met.

Rather than examining the variations among these publicly administered systems, we propose to examine what may be the hardest case to address, the specific form the challenge takes in the United States, hoping that lessons learned here will provide guidance for settings elsewhere. Large American purchasers of health care have increasingly turned to organizations that specialize in providing pharmacy benefit management services to contain rapidly increasing budgets for drugs. Sometimes these services are provided by divisions within large insurers, including large managed care organizations, and sometimes they are provided by separate companies, often called "carve-outs." These organizations promise lower costs as a result of economies of scale that permit manufacturer rebates, retail pharmacy network discounts, efficient mail-order pharmacies, better information systems, capabilities to affect drug utilization, and cost-saving limits on drug benefits. The specific features of the contracts they make reflect the specific goals and demands of the purchasers of the plan—large self-insured employers and large insurance programs. The two largest commercial pharmacy benefit management companies (PBMs) alone manage drug benefits for over 100 million Americans. Millions more of the heaviest users of pharmaceuticals will be added if PBMs are made the vehicle for providing a new Medicare drug benefit.

Are we doomed to repeat the past because we have not learned its lessons? Are we setting administrators of pharmacy benefits up for the same intense backlash in the next decade that managed care more generally faced in the last half of the 1990s? After all, these organizations confront a public informed by the Internet and influenced by direct consumer advertising, an aging population that uses more drugs, dramatic new products, "disease management" strategies that rely on use of the best new treatments, and intense media attention. Pharmacy benefit managers work in a climate in which purchasers fear that rising drug costs will undermine their ability to offer any drug coverage at all. These purchasers put increasing pressure on PBMs, but they largely remain hidden from employee and public view, leaving the PBM to take the heat from patient and physician discontent. Isn't this a formula for repeated failure and increased distrust?

We are not doomed to repeat the past, provided we avoid acting as if the organizations providing pharmacy benefits will create a technical fix for what is at heart a political and ethical problem. Pharmacy benefit managers cannot (and should not) hide the problem of fair limits, any more than managed care more generally can hide it, or any more than "bureaucratic muddling through" can hide it in publicly managed health systems (Daniels 2000; Daniels & Sabin, 2001). Implementing accountability for reasonableness in pharmacy benefit management can address the legitimacy problem that has fueled distrust elsewhere in the health care system. In addition, a Medicare drug benefit that required such accountability would play a significant role in shaping the whole playing field, both public and private, and could provide a model for avoiding the kind of distrust the United States is currently experiencing. Of course, the kind of transparency we advocate here is opposed by those who fear public resistance to limits, but our approach offers the only way to educate clinicians and the public so that, over time, better decisions about limits can be made and accepted as reasonable.

DRUG BUDGETS: PRICES, VOLUME, AND THE SILO PROBLEM

Our argument in what follows depends crucially on having a correct understanding of the causes and implications of the rising cost of pharmacy benefits. We address two objections to our approach before elaborating it.

The first objection is that we are attacking the wrong problem, that we are advocating limiting or rationing needed drugs when we should be challenging big pharmaceutical companies. Many people believe that the real problem regarding drugs and their cost is the pricing policies of large manufacturers, especially as they apply to the U.S. market. They point out that Americans pay extremely high prices for new drugs—much higher than people in many foreign countries pay. If we cut those prices, we would not have a problem of soaring drug costs. The real American policy issue, in this view, is to adopt policies that resemble those of foreign countries, reducing prices by large-scale purchasing or price controls. Minimally, we need full transparency about pricing policies. Otherwise, the huge public investment Americans pay for in the form of basic pharmaceutical research ends up subsidizing health care in other countries while contributing to excessive rates of profits in the United States.

Our reply is that there are *two* problems of drug costs, not one—high domestic prices *and* rapidly rising budgets, and *both* must be addressed. If there were only the problem of excessive prices for new drugs, then reasonable pharmacy limits would not solve it. Pursuing such limits would appropriately be greeted with skepticism, distrust, and outrage, for such limits would take benefits from patients in order to give excessive profits to large corporations. (Just when profits are excessive is a question we cannot address here, but our intuition is that profits are excessive if they are not necessary to produce an appropriate level of investment in drug development. We should not, however, judge what is appropriate by reference to the current level of investment in drug development, since market decisions about drug development are often aimed at providing products for which great demand can be anticipated or created, not by estimates of how to improve population health or meet urgent needs. Thus, we get the marginally improved allergy drug but not the new treatment for malaria. In any case, without greater transparency about pricing policies and development strategies, we cannot address this issue.[2])

Other countries that reduce the prices they pay for drugs through various purchasing strategies and regulatory measures still face the same critical problem Americans face—rapidly rising drug budgets—and they must take steps to address it. Of course, they face the problem at a lower level of cost, which is clearly a gain for them, but they still face the problem of rapidly increasing pressures on drug budgets. If Americans were able to lower domestic drug prices through comparable measures, they would have a substantial, one-time saving in their system. But Americans would still find that, like citizens of other countries, their drug budgets were rising more quickly than other health care budgets. They would still have to address that problem through reasonable pharmacy management.

Though American drug-pricing policies contribute significantly to the high drug budgets we now see, the rate of budget increase is not explained by these pricing policies alone. What is at work in the United States, just as it is in other countries that enforce different pricing policies, is a distinct phenomenon, namely, a set of trends that increase the volume of prescription use and introduce new drugs that are both more effective and more costly. These trends demand proper pharmacy management and accountability for reasonable limits on third-party funding of drugs. Since these trends explain the rapid increase in drug budgets, whether or not drug pricing problems have been addressed in different countries, we believe our proposal about accountability for reasonableness is relevant and important independently of solving the problem of how to balance incentives for research, publicly subsidized research, and drug pricing in the United States.

We shall back up our reasons for this analysis of the rapid rise of pharmacy budgets shortly, but first we want to address the other objection to our approach. Suppose we are right that the main reasons for the rate of increase in pharmacy budgets are trends that increase the volume of prescriptions, including the introduction of new drugs that are often more costly than the ones they replace (i.e., the effects of innovation and increased utilization). It still does not follow that we should be alarmed about pharmacy budget increases and advocate limit setting on pharmaceuticals. If we are buying more health benefit with our drug expenditures, then why limit what we spend? In any case, increases in the drug "silo" may be offset, at least partly, by savings elsewhere in the complex health care granary. If new drugs are more effective, they may reduce hospital admissions, shorten hospital stays, or reduce the need for intensive outpatient or home care, saving money overall, even if they are more costly than older drugs.

This objection raises a sound point, but it is not an objection to what we advocate. The greater effectiveness of new drugs, where it exists, is exactly what reasonable pharmacy management must consider. Similarly, the effects across budgets, or silos, are exactly what must be measured and considered in the reasonable design of a pharmacy benefit. Accountability for reasonableness takes the perspective of the covered population and all stakeholders in cooperative schemes intended to improve population health fairly within reasonable resource limits. It resists the limited perspective of a single silo, but it is not blind to overall limits on resources. Obviously, this means reconciling—with public accountability—the interests of large purchasers (public or private), the populations they buy coverage for, and the health plans and other benefit managers with whom they contract.

We return, then, to consider the reasons why pharmacy budgets are rising at such high rates. It is tempting to point to price inflation; during the 1980s and early 1990s, the public became used to hearing about medical inflation rates much higher than the general rate of inflation. In that vein, one recent study by Families USA points to price increases in the 50 drugs most commonly used by the elderly that are nearly double the general rate of inflation (Pear, 2000), though the general rate of health care inflation also exceeds the general inflation rate.

Most studies, however, suggest that factors other than price inflation are the main sources of pharmacy budget increases in the last decade. First, let's be clear about the levels of budget increase we are considering. During the 1980s, national health expenditures increased about 189%, while drug expenditures increased about 205% (Levit, Cowan, Lazenby, et al., 2000). In contrast, during the 1990s, national health expenditures increased only 97%, in large part due to a significant drop in the middle of the decade when annual increases were 4%–5%, rising to 6%–7% by the end of the decade. Drug expenditures in the 1990s, however, continued to increase at 206%, with annual increases ranging from 11% to 14%–15%. Even the Families USA evidence about drug price inflation only accounts for, at most, one-third of the increased drug budget expenditures.

What other factors are at work? A key factor is a significant increase in the volume of drugs prescribed and used. Our population is aging, and older people use more medical services, including drugs. New products address the chronic illnesses that dominate our disease profile in an aging population. Many of these products are advertised directly to consumers, and information about them is more available to patients and clinicians through advertising and the Internet than ever before.

If we look at key types of drugs contributing to the current trend, such as new drugs for acid-peptic disorders (including "heartburn"), lipid-lowering drugs, anti-inflammatory drugs, antidepressants, and new diabetes treatments, almost invariably, the major factor contributing to costs is an increase in the utilization rate, not inflation in drug prices. For example, one large PBM found a 32% per member cost increase in 1999 in a relatively new class of drugs for treating acid-peptic disorders, but only about one-eighth of that increase was due to price changes in the drug category. More dramatically, also in 1999, a key class of antidepressants, Prozac and its cousins (the "selective serotonin reuptake inhibitors," or SSRIs), showed an 11% increase in per-member costs, but only one-tenth of that was due to price changes. When this PBM examined the 10 drug categories responsible for 53% of the total increased cost trend in the period 1997–1999, in six of the ten categories, utilization changes greatly outweighed cost per day as a factor. The four categories where cost per day was more important than utilization changes accounted for only 15% of the total increase in costs in that period.

Contributing to the increased utilization rates are new indications for existing drugs. Thus antidepressants are now being used for social phobia, premature ejaculation, premenstrual distress disorder and post-traumatic stress syndrome, not just for the depression for which they were originally tested and approved. New drugs, however, constitute 50% of the trend toward cost increase in the last five years, largely because they generally cost more than the drugs they replace. Given the very large numbers of new drugs in the pipeline awaiting approval, and subtracting the patent expirations of important drugs in the next few years, we can expect the cost-increasing trend to continue throughout the foreseeable future.

In short, we see the following pattern of factors driving the trend to higher drug budgets: an aging population, improved treatments from new drugs, new markets for established drugs, increased consumer demand stimulated in part by over \$2 billion a year in drug advertising, and drug price increases. One large PBM quantified an estimate of the contribution of several implications of these combined factors toward increased drug costs: more users would contribute a 4% increase, more days of therapy per user another 5% increase, a more expensive mix of drugs would add 3%, and higher unit costs would add 3%–5%, for a total of 15%–18% projected cost increase. This estimate conforms with another that attributes one-third of the drug cost increase to inflation, another third to greater drug use, and another to the introduction of new, more expensive drugs (Pear, 2000).

These cost-increasing pressures on pharmacy budgets operate in the United States and abroad; they are not simply the results of the design of the American system. Accountability for reasonableness will not provide pharmacy managers with dramatically more powerful approaches for cutting drug budgets in the short run. By contributing, however, to the legitimacy, stability, and acceptability of appropriate limit-setting measures, accountability for reasonableness could help make pharmacy management a more powerful tool in the long run.

ENCOUNTERING THE TOOLBOX USED TO ADMINISTER PHARMACY BENEFITS

Typically, the design of a pharmacy benefit is the result of an agreement between a purchaser of those benefits, such as a large employer, sometimes after negotiation with a union, and an organization that delivers and administers the benefit. Though the PBM may influence and affect coverage limitations set by the purchaser, it is the payer's plan design that sets the coverage limitations. An employee may often hold the PBM accountable for limits, but, ultimately, key limits are the responsibility of the employer (or government agency purchasing the benefit). Our goal is to hold both purchaser and administrators accountable for the reasonableness of the pharmacy benefit.

To understand the tools PBMs use to contain drug budgets, and to see how accountability for reasonableness affects their use, consider what happens when Louise, who suffers from migraine headaches, goes to her retail pharmacist with a prescription for Imitrex.[3] Louise, many will remember, achieved national fame in 1993 when she and her husband Harry appeared in a notorious $15 million insurance-industry-sponsored series of TV ads that attacked the "big government" Clinton health care reform because it would "take away their choices" in health care. Her migraines cannot be attributed to the restricted choices she may have encountered since or to those she is about to encounter in the scenarios that follow.

A little background is necessary. Imitrex belongs to a class of drugs known colloquially as "triptans," first introduced in the mid-1990s as a breakthrough in the treatment of migraines. While these drugs are not much more effective in aborting migraines than other drugs, they are generally better tolerated. Migraine sufferers are up and about sooner than with other drugs. Confident of their value, manufacturers priced these drugs at a premium. Because there are 22 million migraine sufferers in the United States, and because there has been very effective direct advertising to them, these drugs have a significant impact on drug budgets. Since there are currently four comparably effective triptans on the market, large purchasers of drug benefits can take advantage of competition to reduce drug costs. Through discounts (or more problematically, rebates) they can use incentives to direct utilization toward specific drugs that are less expensive for them to buy. In what follows, Louise encounters three tools that PBMs frequently use to administer coverage limitations set by the plan design selected by the purchasers.

Scenario 1: Louise and Prior Authorization

When Louise presents her prescription for Imitrex to the druggist at her local pharmacy, he enters it in his computer. The automated adjudication program tells him that Louise's benefit plan requires "prior authorization" for triptans. He explains that prior authorization is a process used to determine if coverage conditions are met when more information is needed than is available from the prescription or from the claim information provided by the pharmacy. He apologizes, deftly deflects her annoyance, and gives her a 1-800 phone number to initiate the process.

From the drugstore, Louise calls the 800-number and is told that her doctor will be contacted immediately to get the additional information needed to determine coverage eligibility. Worried that a delay might leave her vulnerable to an untreated migraine, Louise says that she has tried various painkillers, which do not help, and that the doctor has assured her she will do better with Imitrex. Doesn't the doctor, she asks, know what she needs?

Louise has a good question. Doesn't her doctor know what is best for her? Why require a bureaucratic procedure that annoys both doctor and patient?

Critics believe that these mechanisms ration via the hassle factor, and that the only reason for the hassle is cost. There are, however, two possible justifications or rationales for the requirement. One rationale is that the plan contracts to pay for drugs, including triptans, only when they are being safely and effectively used. Triptans are effective for aborting migraines, not for preventing them, yet many patients who demand them from doctors hope to avoid ever having migraines again. Triptans are also potentially dangerous for some uses.

This reason could be (but need not be) interpreted as a challenge to the competency of the doctor, or even as a way to coerce compliance with a guideline for the use of a drug. Such an interpretation seems to demand additional, relevant evidence: do doctors have inappropriate patterns of prescription for this class of drugs in the absence of prior authorization? Without such evidence, challenging the doctor seems unwarranted or gratuitous. And if the plan has good pharmaceutical reason to encourage a specific pattern of prescription, then it generally does so by sending recommendations directly to physicians, who have to be persuaded of the rationale for the change. There may be, however, a more benign interpretation of this reason for prior authorization, namely that the plan has no obligation to pay for specific unsafe or ineffective uses of drugs that it can identify.

The second potential rationale for prior authorization is, in any case, the primary one: for many patients, less expensive migraine remedies will actually work quite well. The savings that come from not using triptans as a first line of response are significant and can help to make resources available for expensive drugs when they are truly necessary. A patient who does not do well with other remedies will be covered for triptans. A patient who cannot take other remedies, for example, because of allergy or other contraindications to them, can be exempted from the restriction. The second reason is thus a concern for the stewardship of resources.

What should be said to a patient who replies, "I don't care about conserving resources, I want the best medicine for my problem?" If a less expensive medicine safely and effectively aborts migraines for a patient, there may be no basis for saying that the triptan is the "best medicine" for that patient. When a less expensive treatment does not manage the problem well for a particular patient, or cannot be used, as in the case of contraindications, then the triptan will be covered. It is often the case that when a patient has been taking a drug such as a triptan, and a new pharmacy benefit plan is introduced that requires prior authorization for it, the use is "grandfathered in" to avoid the protest that would come from disrupting an established, effective treatment (even if another might work as well).

We believe the second rationale for prior authorization is one that fair-minded patients and clinicians should accept as relevant and reasonable, even if they do not like the consequences in a particular case. Given an efficient procedure for appealing the restriction for specific patients, let us suppose the prior authorization can meet all the requirements for accountability for reasonableness. This still leaves the important question of how and when should Louise be made aware of the rationale.

Ideally, the physician could be given fingertip access to the patient's benefit restrictions on triptans through his own office-based computer system or through a Palm Pilot that provides integrated access to the features of all available plans. Doctors complain vigorously about the flood of advisories sent by the provider or the administrator of the pharmacy benefits, and many pay no attention to them since they often provide information when it is not needed. Whether new technologies can be provided to reduce the physician burden in adjusting to the features of a patient's benefit restrictions remains an open question. Without some technological assistance, however, time pressures on physicians—the result of increased workloads under cost containment pressures—work against using even such immediate access. Prior authorization is only infrequently used in administering pharmacy benefits—only a couple of dozen drugs may reasonably invoke it, for example, because some of their uses are covered and others not. Physicians who deal with a small number of plans frequently become aware of their rules. If Louise's physician had been aware of the restriction, he could have alerted her to it and avoided her annoyance when she discovered it at the point of sale. The pharmacist might also have had in his computer access to the rationales—and even the evidentiary base—for various restrictions.

It might also be possible for Louise to receive an explanation of the rationale when she calls the 1–800 number to initiate the procedure. In some plans, this is primarily viewed as a clerical step. In others, a pharmacist receives the call and could provide a rationale for it. Proper training and properly designed computer programs could give such a pharmacist immediate access to a rationale, including evidence where it plays a role in the restriction. Finally, Louise should have access to rationales for important restrictions the PBM uses through literature aimed at enrollees and through a website structured to explain, to the level of detail requested, the grounds for features of the benefit design.

Scenario 2: Louise and the Tiered Co-payment Benefit Structure

When Louise gives her prescription for Imitrex to her druggist, his computer tells him that Imitrex requires a $30 co-pay, the highest of three co-pay levels in her tiered co-payment benefit structure. Had her physician prescribed Zomig, another drug in the same class, she would only have a $15 co-pay. (Were there a generic drug in this class, she could have it for $10.) She complains that she has tried Zomig and found it not very effective. Why should she have to pay more?

In fact, Louise should not have to pay more in this case, but let us first understand why PBMs use tiered co-payment plans. The primary reason for tiering is to provide incentives to the patient to accept the least expensive drug that is likely to be effective for her. A preference for a nongeneric, when there is an appropriate, good quality, generic alternative, will then cost the patient an additional amount. The middle tier will contain a "preferred" brand, in this case Zomig, whereas the nonpreferred brand will cost an even higher co-pay. In some plans, the co-pay for the nonpreferred brand may be some percentage of the drug cost, leading to even higher costs for the patient.

Drugs are selected for the middle tier primarily on the basis of price among those drugs or drug classes that are generally interchangeable on clinical grounds. If one triptan—say Zomig—can by bought by the purchaser (through the benefit manager) at a substantial discount, then it is likely to be used more often than drugs with higher co-pays. If competition then forces other companies to provide comparable discounts, more drugs might end up in the middle category. Where competing drugs are of equivalent effectiveness, and are equally free of side effects, then the rationale for the tiering seems unproblematic. Where, however, a patient can tolerate a nonpreferred drug better than a preferred one, or where the nonpreferred drug is clearly more effective for a particular patient, it is generally unfair to impose a higher cost on the patient. It is at this point that a clinician should be able to appeal the pricing of the tiers and secure a lower co-pay for the patient. Louise falls into this category.

More problematic is the case when the middle-tier drugs are generally not quite as effective or have more negative side effects than the nonpreferred drug. A drug that was slightly more effective or had slightly fewer side effects might not be discounted, even if it ended up in the higher tier, because the manufacturer would be confident that patient and clinician demand for it would remain high. In this case, the middle tier represents the judgment that the treatment is clinically good enough and that, if a patient wants better than that, it is justifiable to shift costs to her.

For this rationale to constitute a reason fair-minded people (that is, those who seek mutually justifiable terms of cooperation) can accept as relevant, people would have to be persuaded that the "clinically good enough" is truly good enough and that the extra benefits of the higher tier are those we have less obligation to provide for each other. Where reasonable people think that the burdens that the merely good enough impose are ones we owe it to each other to reduce, they would not find the tiering acceptable. There will be tension between an employer who is only interested in what is good enough to retain employees and the employees and their clinicians who are concerned about what is clinically good enough. This tension can best be addressed by open deliberation about the fair terms of cooperation in this situation.

This problematic case leads to a more general point about co-pays. Co-pays shift costs to patients in need of drugs. When is such cost-shifting justifiable? Where co-pays provide an incentive to use cheaper but equivalent drugs, shifting some cost to patients seems a justifiable way of introducing incentives to conserve collective resources. Where co-pays play a role in reducing unnecessary use of some drugs, the cost-shifting they involve also seems a reason all can accept. The case involving the judgment that some drugs are good enough is problematic just because reasonable people would have to agree that the scarcity is severe enough to limit our obligations to each other in this way.

A key assumption underlies the rationale provided for tiering, namely that the lower price of drugs that become "preferred" brands are the results of discounts to the purchaser, and that the savings from these discounts are available to provide sustainable benefits to the patient population. If, however, we are concerned with rebates (to the purchaser or the PBM) and not discounts, that is, with payments to the organizations administering the benefits that directly contribute to their profits, then we are in murky waters. Patients and clinicians will be suspicious that the pharmacy benefit provider—the employer—and PBM administrator are together in a conflict of interest in which they may be imposing burdens on the patient population for their own gain. A public that accepts the idea of for-profit delivery systems, believing, correctly or not, that competition among plans yields both good care and value for money, will plausibly insist that there is a difference between a rebate and a discount, that rebates smell of corruption, especially if they are not transparent, whereas all can understand a discount. Obviously, transparency about pricing policies would be important in eliminating distrust and focusing on choices that those affected by them can agree meet population needs fairly under cost constraints.

Let us return to Louise, who has complained about the higher co-pay. If, as she claims, Zomig does not work for her, it does seem unfair to shift more costs to her simply because Zomig has been made the preferred drug for reasons of price. (This is not a case where Zomig is "clinically good enough" but Louise wants "better," which, in any case, is often clearer conceptually than clinically.) A plan that was accountable for reasonableness would provide a readily accessible path for Louise's doctor to appeal the co-pay. In addition, the rationale for the tiering should be accessible to Louise through several paths—her pharmacist's computer, literature sent to her, a website available to her or her clinician, or a 1–800 number where a pharmacist would have fingertip access to a detailed rationale for the features of the plan that affect her co-pays.

Scenario 3: Louise and Limits on Quantity

The prescription Louise hands her druggist is for enough Imitrex to treat six migraines. The pharmacist is notified through his automated claims adjudication program that the maximum quantity covered for a 30-day period is enough Imitrex to treat four migraines. He fills her prescription, but with only enough tablets to treat four migraines (at maximum dose), and he informs Louise of the difference. Louise is angry because she often experiences up to six migraines in a month. The druggist gives her a phone number that she can use if the quantity covered turns out to be insufficient.

Impatient, Louise phones to appeal the limit, fearing that if she waits till her allotment is exhausted, she may end up with no remedy for the next migraine. When she calls, a pharmacist explains that four treatments are sufficient for most patients, and that is why the limit has been imposed. He also says that she can obtain more pills only if prophylactic remedies are also tried. She will have to obtain a prescription for a preventative remedy if she has not already tried one. The PBM pharmacist then phones Louise's physician and explains the requirement to her. A prophylactic remedy is then prescribed as well.

Louise and the clinician resent the nuisance of the quantity restriction, but if preventive measures are effective, Louise may not need the additional, more expensive, abortive treatments. If prevention does not work, her future prescriptions will be adjusted so that she need not appeal the quantity limit again. Quantity limits have two effects: they may reduce the waste that comes with over-prescription, and, because of co-pays, they shift more costs to patients. Such cost shifting may save the pharmacy benefit payer (e.g., the employer) and (if there is risk sharing) the benefit administrator money, but it does not really reduce health care costs.

As in the other scenarios, if the physician had fingertip, in-office access to the patient's benefit structure and how it applied to this prescription, she might have been able to avoid Louise discovering the limit on quantity at the point of sale. She might have prescribed the preventive treatment right away, or appealed the limit directly. Were the computer linkage sophisticated enough, the rationale for the restriction could have been supplied to the physician and Louise in the doctor's office. The value of having the rationales—and not simply rules—at whatever point Louise encounters the limit, whether in the doctor's office or the drug store, is that they can be educative about the importance of conserving resources and they can reveal a pattern of thoughtful attempts to meet needs fairly under budget constraints. And, via the Revision and Appeals Condition, they can facilitate improved policies via the give-and-take of deliberation and debate.

The most common objection to the approach we have described here is that it places unrealistic burdens on both patients and physicians to be aware of and adjust to detailed features of benefit plans. In the United States the presence of multiple competing plans, each with its own protocol, adds an additional layer of complexity and burden. It will be difficult to overcome this objection without better information systems that lighten the burden on physicians, pharmacists, and patients, and it is likely that such systems will only become available through cooperation among large PBMs or systems administrators. It might seem, then, that our strategy here relies on a technological fix. There is no doubt that new information technology will help. The main thrust of our proposal, however, is educational, not technological. Physicians, pharmacists, and patients, as well as purchasers and managers, must become better educated about reasonable limits for drugs. The incentive to produce that education, and the technologies that will facilitate it, derives from the failure of any approach that ducks the problem of changing our understanding and, through it, our motivation to cooperate.

AN "ETHICAL TEMPLATE" FOR PHARMACY BENEFITS

The educational task can be simplified by constructing an "ethical template" for the design of formularies and pharmacy benefits more generally. The template maps resource allocation decisions at different levels of specificity within a typical pharmacy benefit onto rationales that fair-minded people could agree are relevant to meeting pharmacy needs under resource constraints. By involving groups of stakeholders in a process of testing the acceptability of these rationales and in refining the template, greater clarity will result about what counts as reasonable rationales in this domain.

The design of a drug formulary—a list of those drugs that will be covered by a pharmacy benefit—can serve as an paradigm for a pharmacy insurance. Some pharmacy benefit programs contain no formulary limits and rely on patient cost sharing as the control factor, but many public and private benefits incorporate a formulary that embodies various limit-setting decisions. We can think of such a formulary as the result of a hierarchical process of decisions about access to drugs.

Limits in a formulary are set at four basic levels: the categories of drugs that will be included, the selection of drugs within these categories, the specifications for the conditions for use of the selected drugs, and further limits on the amount of drugs to be made available or how they should be obtained (for example, by mail order or in specific pharmacies). These limits can become the basis for levels of patient cost sharing in an actual benefit. We saw these features emerging in Louise's encounter with her benefits.

Different kinds of reasons or rationales play a prominent role at the different levels. For example, at the level of drug categories to be covered, we generally see broad rationales such as: inclusion of drugs that treat "pathology" and exclusion of those that "enhance" otherwise normal traits, inclusion of proven therapies and exclusion of those that are experimental, inclusion of therapies shown to be safe and effective and exclusion of those that are not, and some considerations of cost-worthiness. If we examine the categories that are currently excluded by large, private purchasers of pharmacy benefits, however, we may find a confusing mix of reasons and exclusions. Smoking deterrents, obesity treatments, or even cholesterol-lowering drugs may not be covered because the economic benefits of prevention may not occur to the payer. This shows a clear divergence between a societal perspective on benefit and that of an individual employer buying a pharmacy benefit for a workforce that may have high turnover. Sometimes exclusions, such as for infertility drugs or drugs for erectile dysfunction, are excluded as lifestyle choices that are not the responsibility of the purchaser.

Once the categories of drugs that will be covered are determined—preferably by an appeal to reasons fair-minded people would consider reasonable and properly applied—particular drugs are selected. At this level, the primary driver of decision-making is a balance between meeting patient needs and cost-savings. In some drug categories, a number of drugs will be seen as "generally therapeutically interchangeable"—meaning that they provide the same therapeutic benefits for most people under most conditions. Where there truly is such interchangeability better discounts or rebates may be achieved by offering a manufacturer a favored position in the formulary, thus giving a drug a clear cost-advantage over comparable drugs. Arguably, it is then in the interest of all stakeholders to permit the use of such cost-advantage as a reason for preferred position in the formulary. Allowing this consideration, however, presupposes that there is a clear basis in evidence for interchangeability and that patients for whom there is reason to believe that the preferred drugs fail have a readily available exception process that allows them to be treated appropriately.

As we descend to the next level in the hierarchy to consider limits on the conditions that selected drugs may be used for, a broader range of rationales again appears, similar to the range of rationales applied in making decisions about categories of drugs. For example, retin-A can be used to treat severe acne. This use is covered in most formularies, but the same drug can be used for cosmetic treatment of wrinkles of aging, which is generally not covered. A drug for treating symptoms of Alzheimer's may be covered for mild and moderate forms of the disease, but excluded for severe forms of dementia, when effectiveness has not been established or it has been shown to be ineffective. And, a drug that offers some greater advantage in avoiding side effects, but at a much greater cost, may be excluded or covered at a higher cost-share, unless the less expensive alternatives fail to work for a given patient.

Finally, formularies may set restrictions on drug use even for indications that are covered, as we saw with Louise, who encountered a limit on how many tablets would be covered per month. The primary reason for these restrictions is cost control. Similarly, restrictions on how the drug may be obtained—by mail or through specific retail outlets—would be for cost reasons. To be persuasive to patients and physicians, the cost rationale must appeal to collective gain that results from the savings. There may have to be some explanation of how the savings arise and how the benefit from them will be used, such as by lowering premiums, broadening coverage, or sustaining coverage despite an overall rise in drug costs.

An ethical template would map reasons that different stakeholders agree are relevant onto the types of decisions made at different levels. It would then serve as a guide—but not a blueprint—for decision-making. Relevant reasons can be given different weights. The template determines a range of acceptable benefits, not a single uniquely fair pharmacy benefit. It provides a guide in the form of types of relevant reasons that can facilitate making rationales public and fully transparent. It requires a readily available process for appeals, exceptions, and revision over time, thus meeting the third condition of accountability for reasonableness.

A properly developed ethical template will inform whatever educational process is developed for making physicians, patients, and pharmacists aware of the limits to pharmacy benefits. Education can be about options, the evidence for them, and the ethical rationales. The template provides a common language for further debate and deliberation about pharmacy coverage. In this way, the template helps accountability for reasonableness teach us as a society how to share pharmacy resources.

HARRY AND LOUISE GROW UP

LOUISE (Entering with packages): Harry, I'm home.

HARRY (In front of the TV): Did you get your pills?

LOUISE: Yes, but you won't believe the hassle. I was only able to get four doses—but Dr. Frank had ordered more.

HARRY: The druggist wouldn't give you what he ordered?

LOUISE: Your drug plan—they have rules.

HARRY: Who made them boss? They're not our doctor. I told you years ago they would ruin our health care.

LOUISE: No, Harry, you said it was the government. But this is your health plan.

HARRY: I guess it's all the same.

LOUISE: You know, I've been thinking. They gave me reasons why they have those rules, and they weren't all nonsense. I can see how they have to hold costs down. At least we have drugs covered. Remember how Mom didn't when she was very sick in those last months? They cost a lot, and she would take fewer to save money.

HARRY: Yeah, I remember.

LOUISE: If we retire in a couple of years, we'll be doing just what she did.

HARRY: Maybe not. They're talking about Medicare paying for drugs.

LOUISE: Now you want the government interfering!

HARRY: Not interfering, paying.

LOUISE: Well, you can't have both. If they're going to pay, they'll make rules, just like your company does. So long as the rules make sense.

NOTES

1. We wish to thank Russell Teagarden for extensive help in preparing this chapter.

2. Just how to balance public interests and private incentives is a difficult policy issue that requires careful thought about how to assign private property rights in technologies that build on publicly funded research and careful public examination of generally proprietary information about drug development strategies and costs employed by pharmaceutical companies. We refrain from speculation on them here.

3. Scenarios in this section were provided by Russell Teagarden, Vice President for Clinical Practices and Therapeutics at Merck Medco Managed Care.

8

INDIRECT LIMIT SETTING: ACCOUNTABILITY FOR PHYSICIAN INCENTIVES

Primacy of Patient Welfare over Physician's Financial Interests
Under no circumstances may physicians place their own financial
interests above the welfare of their patients. The primary objective
of the medical profession is to render service to humanity; reward
or financial gain is a subordinate consideration. For a physician
unnecessarily to hospitalize a patient, prescribe a drug, or conduct
diagnostic tests for the physician's financial benefit is unethical.
Similarly to limit appropriate diagnostic tests, referrals, hospitaliza-
tions, or treatments for the physician's financial benefit is unethical.
If a conflict develops between the physician's financial interests and
the physician's responsibilities to the patient, the conflict must be
resolved to the patient's benefit.[1]

PUBLIC ACCOUNTABILITY FOR A SOCIAL EXPERIMENT

We have illustrated what accountability for reasonableness requires in several
areas of direct limit setting by health plans or public agencies, such as coverage
for new technologies, management of last-chance therapies, and limits on pharmacy benefits. But much of the limit setting carried out in the United States is indirect, not direct. It depends on giving incentives to physicians to alter their practice patterns in cost-conscious ways. Experiments in a similar direction have been
undertaken in the British National Health Service (NHS), where physician groups
have been made "fundholders" for their patients.

If capitation schemes and other incentives to physicians were clinical trials of
new methods or decision procedures for treating an illness, they would be submitted to Institutional Review Boards for review and approval. Such boards are
charged with evaluating all experimentation on human subjects. Any risks imposed by incentive schemes that reasonable persons would want to know about
would have to be discussed fully in securing informed consent from the human
subjects—in this case, all insured patients.

Although the new incentives aim at changing clinical decisions, and presumably
succeed at doing so, they are not subject to these methods of public accountabil-

ity. There is no public accountability for them even though the incentives also pose novel conflicts of interest with the Primacy Principle (cited above) and thus threaten trust in doctors. The health system is conducting an unregulated social experiment.

To introduce public accountability into this experiment, we pose the following touchstone question to physicians and health plans: Do you have arguments and evidence that should persuade fair-minded persons that the financial incentives you apply are a reasonable limit-setting device and pose no undue risks to patients or the Primacy Principle? Posed this way, the touchstone question is a special application of the Publicity and Relevance Conditions discussed in Chapter 4.

When physicians decide which of the myriad risks and benefits associated with a proposed treatment they should inform their patients about, they often use the device of asking themselves what a "reasonable" patient would want to know. In similar fashion, the device of the "fair-minded" patient (see Chapter 4) focuses accountability on reasons relevant to justifying the incentives. Just as we can think of informed consent as an essential component of collaborative planning of treatments or clinical trials, so too, answering the touchstone question engages patients and the public in collaborative deliberation about rules of delivering health care that all can agree are reasonable. Holding plans and physicians publicly accountable for answering this question about the reasonableness of incentives is crucial to establishing their legitimate authority to conduct this clinical trial on the doctor-patient relationship.

After distinguishing empirical questions about trust ("Have the new incentives eroded trust?") from the normative question that is our concern here ("Should patients trust physicians working under these incentives?"), we argue that neither reaffirmations of the Primacy Principle ("Trust us.") nor simple disclosure of conflicts of interest will assure us that we should trust physicians who accept certain incentives. Satisfying existing guidelines for the design of incentives might allay concerns about trust, but these guidelines rest on theoretical considerations and are not yet supported by evidence about the actual effects of these schemes. Accountability for reasonableness requires such evidence. If health plans provide such evidence, and physicians are prepared to present it, then it will strengthen the institutional support for physicians' ethical obligations. Unfortunately, meeting this demand for evidence about the safety and effects of reimbursement schemes is difficult. The studies needed to produce this information have not been done and would be difficult and expensive to design and conduct. In the course of this chapter, we will evaluate what this means for accountability for reasonableness.

THE THREAT TO TRUST

As large purchasers have intensified their efforts to contain health care costs through the spread of managed care, more and more physicians have agreed to work under financial incentives aimed at limiting care and its overall cost. Most commonly, the health plan "withholds" some percentage of the income of an otherwise fee-for-service provider, restoring the "withhold" if organizational cost targets are achieved (Gold, Hurley, Lake et al., 1995). With increasing frequency, physician groups, often those with the least familiarity with the cost-conscious culture of traditional prepaid group practices like Kaiser Permanente, accept the insurance risk of providing some range of patient services within a negotiated payment per patient per month (Kuttner, 1998). This capitation can also be coupled with bonuses and other incentives to reduce costs or achieve certain quality goals (Bodenheimer & Grumbach, 1996).

These novel incentives are deliberately aimed at changing traditional patterns of clinical decision-making. As the Primacy Principle cited above makes clear, they replace a fee-for-service conflict of interest that encourages physicians to overtreat with one that risks undertreatment (Woolhandler & Himmelstein, 1995). Ideally, they will only induce physicians to avoid unnecessary care and to select appropriate care that is more cost-effective, producing a win-win-win outcome for patients, providers, and purchasers.

But ideals are hard to achieve, and the unknown risk to patients is that appropriate care will be withheld because physicians will put their financial interests above patient needs. This unknown risk replaces the risk of overtreatment from the opposite danger. We need not suppose that overt greed or corruption must underlie this risk. Physicians may perceive or intend no violation of the Primacy Principle and yet violate it, because there is plenty of room for uncertainty, reasonable disagreement, and even self-deception.

Recent studies suggest that, although some physicians embrace the lucrative possibilities capitation can offer (Murray, 1997), many are concerned about the impact of the new incentive structures on their relationships with patients. In a focus-group study in a high-penetration managed care market, physicians expressed concern that their "patients believe that economic forces unduly influence physicians' decisions (Jecker & Jonsen, 1997)." In a broader survey of primary care physicians, doctors believed that capitated care for patients "threatened relationships with patients" and was "costly" to that relationship (Cykert, Hanson, Layson & Joines, 1997). By the mid-1990s, surveys of public and patient attitudes toward managed care showed that approval of physicians was lower than years ago, but still quite high, and much higher than approval of health plans (Miller & Luft, 1997; Knickman, Hughes, Taylor et al., 1996). Of course, media attention to "signal cases" might produce more rapid erosion of confidence in physicians (Johnsson, 1996).

Even if trust in physicians has not yet significantly eroded, these incentives and other changes in the design of our system undercut the authority of physicians by threatening traditional bases for trust (Mechanic, 1997b; Gray, 1997). Mechanic and Schlesinger (1996) propose some steps aimed at rebuilding that trust, for example, by limiting the amount at risk through these incentives, by having plans, rather than physicians, disclose incentive arrangements (which satisfies AMA guidelines), and by having physicians play a visible role of advocate for patients and against health plan coverage limitations.

However effective this strategy for managing distrust may be, it ignores a fundamental normative question: *Should* patients trust physicians with these incentives?

"TRUST US," DISCLOSURE, AND THE PRIMACY PRINCIPLE

Reaffirmation of the Primacy Principle and simple disclosure of incentives will not suffice in lieu of answering the touchstone question. Physicians cannot just say, "It doesn't matter what the reimbursement scheme is, we know in our hearts what appropriate patient care is, and we will never compromise it because of our financial or career interests." Obviously, physicians can't simply say this if patients have already lost trust in them. Even if patients still generally do trust their doctors, they and we both should know that incentives do change physician behavior.

We know, for example, that reducing reimbursement rates to physicians in fee-for-service arrangements under Medicare in the 1970s and 1980s led to their increasing the quantity and intensity of services they provided (Rice, 1997)—with unknown effects on patients. Nor is it only market-oriented American physicians who respond to incentives: by adding some fee-for-service incentives for specific, underutilized services, the Danes were able to alter physician decisions (Karasnik, Groenewegen, Pedersen et al., 1990).

More to the point, there is a growing body of evidence about the responsiveness of physicians to incentives aimed at limiting care and its cost. Compared to physicians under fee-for-service indemnity insurance, primary care physicians under salary, and even more so those under capitation, reduce their hospitalization rates and their rates of referral to specialists (Stearns, Wolfe, & Kindig, 1992; Hillman, Pauly, & Kerstein, 1989). Capitated specialty groups, such as radiologists, cardiologists, and obstetricians and gynecologists, as well as dentists, show changes in utilization patterns of various services. There is evidence that physicians react to cost incentives most strongly where there is the most uncertainty about how to treat, as reflected in areas that have the greatest variation in physician practice, such as asthma, dehydration, seizures, pneumonia or urinary tract infection (Josephson & Karcz, 1997). Thus, capitated primary care physicians in a for-profit group, as compared to physicians paid on a fee-for-service significantly reduced hospitalization rates and emergency department rates for patients aged 25–44 who had these conditions.

Because this study did not examine patient outcomes, we do not know whether the patients of capitated physicians were at greater risk from the reduced hospitalization rates (the lower emergency department rates were explained by off-hours services provided by the capitated group). It is tempting to conclude that there was no greater risk to them because there are many studies showing no over-all pattern of worse outcomes for patients in capitated plans as opposed to fee-for-service indemnity plans (Berwick, 1996; Cangialose, Cary, Hoffman & Ballard, 1997), despite the fact that the cost-savings in capitated plans derives largely from the incentives they offer to doctors (Hellinger, 1996; Orentlicher, 1996). But this inference is unwarranted since the reimbursement methods used in capitated plans vary widely, and many factors can hide or compensate for the possibly negative effects of capitating physicians directly.

The issue in this study is quite general, since there is similar uncertainty in many medical contexts about whether a test or a referral or a procedure is needed. If incentives incline more and more physicians to resolve uncertainty in favor of imposing more risk on patients, then standards of care will shift. But if the standard of care shifts, the conflict of interest for the practitioner dissolves. Practitioners can honestly affirm their adherence to the Primacy Principle, which only holds them to avoid compromising the standards of care.

Nevertheless, a reasonable worry for patients remains: Do the incentives unduly compromise the standard of care?

It will not do simply to *disclose* the general features of the reimbursement schemes. To be sure, simple disclosure has at least this much to be said for it: although it does not avoid a conflict of interest, it avoids hiding one. Being open about it thus warns all parties to be alert. In effect, disclosure by physicians or health plans says, "Since we are not hiding these incentives, you should trust us not to violate the Primacy Principle."

Even more can be said on behalf of simple disclosure. Disclosure by physicians imposes a kind of "smell test" that would be missing if it were only plans that disclosed incentives. If physicians would be so uncomfortable with the very attempt to explain their method of reimbursement, then it may be because they believe no consumer will like the way it smells. They must suspect it fails to be *reasonable* in the appropriate sense. Still, this smell test turns on physicians' unexamined sensitivities. That is inadequate. How good, after all, is their sense of smell?

Simple disclosure, especially if we think of a disclosure by the health plan that the physician can simply refer to, can also be thought of as a form of market accountability and not as a way of appealing for trust. Patients (consumers) who are informed about alternative reimbursement schemes can, in theory, choose among them, exiting from plans whose schemes they do not like in favor of ones they prefer. According to the market accountability view, this exercise of choice then confers legitimacy, since we consent to the limits of what we buy. In effect, the moral authority rests with us as informed consumers, and it is exercised through our choices.

The simple appeal of this view of market legitimacy is also its downfall, certainly in practice and arguably in theory, as we argued in Chapter 3. In the United States, half of all employees have no choice among health plans. Even those who do have choices among plans cannot "exit" or switch easily once they are ill, which is when they discover in detail how limit-setting structures work. In addition, we have no assurance that a market will generate reasonable limit-setting structures that provide people with appropriate alternatives. Market failure to provide such alternatives—which we can know about only if there is public accountability for the content of these arrangements—invites public intervention.

In reassuring us about incentives, then, physicians (and plans) cannot simply say "Trust us," and they cannot rely on simple disclosure. Instead, they must be prepared to answer our touchstone question.

ACCOUNTABILITY FOR THE REASONABLENESS OF INCENTIVES

Let us return to our touchstone question: Do physicians have arguments that should persuade *fair-minded persons* that these incentive schemes are *reasonable* ways to encourage appropriate limits in cooperative schemes to deliver health care? We do not mean that the whole burden of accountability for reasonableness falls on physicians and the discussions they have with patients, though we take seriously the idea of such conversations. Rather, the device of the touchstone question is intended to clarify what accountability for reasonableness involves wherever decisions about the design and implementation of reimbursement schemes is at issue.

We can illustrate this test of reasonableness by considering another reason why simple disclosure of physician incentives inadequately addresses the problem of conflict of interest and the normative question about trust. If the only problem we face is identifying a hidden conflict of interest, then simple disclosure has some plausibility. But the real problem is more complex.

The real problem involves finding incentives that properly align and balance the several interests that are at stake in cooperative schemes to deliver health care. For example, because we are concerned about population health as well as the health of individual patients, we must consider the interests of all parties in the covered population. Doctors cannot ignore the issue of population health, since they ration their own time and often must make implicit comparisons among their own patients, as when they decide to spend more time with Ms. Smith than with Mr. Jones. Directly to the point, a Canadian physician we interviewed told us he could not overstate the urgency of a patient's condition in order to secure the patient a quicker CT scan because he would no longer be credible in the eyes of the physicians guarding the CT scan and his other patients would suffer. Similarly, a British physician told us of a seminar in which one physician spoke with pride about how he moved his patients higher on the waiting list for surgery. Another physician commented, "In other words, you are pushing my patients lower on the list!"

In addition to conflicts between individual and population health, the private organizations, including for-profits, that organize and deliver care in our system acquire their own interests. These interests may also conflict with the interests of the covered populations as well as with the interests of the physicians that contract with them.

A reimbursement method such as capitation must achieve an appropriate, reasonable balance among these competing interests. This balance must seem reasonable to fair-minded parties cooperating in these schemes in light of their common goal of meeting the health care needs of a covered population fairly under reasonable resource constraints. One implication is that fair-minded parties should recognize a collective interest in pursuing the cost-effective delivery of services. They should recognize that reasonable resource constraints preclude providing every beneficial service regardless of cost, as we argued in Chapter 2.

If cost-effectiveness is relevant to pursuing population goals in health care, then incentives that encourage physicians to think about cost-effectiveness will align their interests with the covered population. At the same time, however, the incentives may involve a conflict of interest with individual patients. Where multiple interests are at stake, the perception of conflict depends on perspective.

Of course, the economic incentives to physicians to undertreat could be too strong. This situation would come about if physicians and health plans form an alliance to share the benefits of reducing costs without careful consideration of the interests of individual patients and the covered population. Physician interests would then conflict both with those of their individual patients and those of the population of patients as a whole.

A reasonable reimbursement method, then, must solve a complex problem in which interests may conflict in several directions. A reasonable solution should not, however, simply be the result of bargaining that reflects the relative power of the different interests. Nor is it reasonable not to have patients at the table. A solution must be based on a consideration of how to achieve the common goal shared by fair-minded parties in providing the best possible care to individuals and the covered population within reasonable resource limits. At least, that is the point behind our touchstone question.

EVALUATING THE REASONABLENESS
OF CAPITATION SCHEMES

So far, the answer to the touchstone question is that fair-minded persons should agree that incentives aimed at inducing physicians to seek cost-effective care are reasonable provided they do not induce inappropriate undertreatment and the violation of the Primacy Principle. Accountability for the reasonableness of incentives now requires plans and physicians to show that this proviso is satisfied. Ideally, showing it is satisfied in the case of a specific incentive scheme would involve giving evidence that the incentives promote the desired goals and do not induce inappropriate care, just as giving evidence about outcomes satisfies expectations of disclosure and informed consent for treatment recommendations. This evidence could take the more indirect form of showing that a particular incentive scheme falls within general guidelines for incentives, where the guidelines are supported by evidence that they protect against inappropriate care.

Unfortunately, there is little in the way of direct, empirical evidence to support the reasonableness of the guidelines that have so far been proposed for the design of incentive systems. For example, an often cited study of the effects of the intensity of incentives (the amount of physician income that is at risk in an incentive system) rests entirely on a survey of health plan managers' judgments about when incentives have an effect and when the level of that effect is "of concern" to the manager because it might lead to inappropriate care (Hillman, Pauly, Kerman, & Martinek, 1991). Few managers surveyed thought incentives below 5% of income were likely to produce noticeable effects; most thought that incentives in the 15%– 30% range would produce noticeable effects on practice, and an increasing number became "concerned" about the effect at the higher end of that range and above it. As the authors of that study noted, however, the judgments of concern are subjective, and physicians other than managers might have quite different judgments about concern. There may be other proprietary evidence about incentives and their effects, but they are not available in the literature and therefore cannot play a role in public accountability for the reasonableness of incentive schemes. Clearly, direct studies are needed.

When HCFA established rules for plans it would reimburse, it required plans with patient panels of less than 25,000 to put no more than 25% of physician income at risk. Larger panels are thought to spread risk adequately and need involve no specific limit on physician income at risk. The HCFA rule, however, even if it fits within the range of judgments that managers' generally feel comfortable with, does not rest on any direct study of incentive effects.

The very absence of direct studies about the effects of reimbursement systems on patient safety and the fact that private and public insurers "fly by the seat of their pants" on this crucial question should raise eyebrows, if not alarm flags. The absence of direct studies is, at least in part, explained by the difficulty of designing and conducting them. One problem such studies face is having a clear measure of what constitutes patient safety. A well-designed study would have to specify just what would count as good and bad outcomes. A second problem is raised by the fact that a study would have to compare the rates of such outcomes to alternative schemes. After all, fee-for-service incentives can induce overtreatment and carry alternative risks. But as new reimbursement systems have driven old ones out of existence, comparisons have become harder to obtain, and they are, in any case, difficult to disentangle from well-known variations in practice patterns. There is also the difficulty of obtaining a large enough base of integrated data on patient outcomes that is linked to specific physicians or groups of physicians so that the correlation between reimbursement features and patient outcomes can be established. Finally, the fact that most physicians treat patients covered by more than one reimbursement scheme makes it difficult to detect the effects of any one scheme. Because of the many variables involved, large studies are necessary to disentangle effects.

These practical problems are serious. The absence of adequate funding for health services research makes them even more so. Still, accountability for the reasonableness of the social experiment involving new reimbursement schemes does mean that the burden is on public and private insurers and providers who use them to offer at least some relevant evidence that can be used in answering our touchstone questions.

In the absence of relevant evidence, we must fall back to the vague and somewhat unsatisfying ethical guidelines that have been advanced. We will consider one proposal that provides a comprehensive analytic framework, but we emphasize from the start that the plausibility of the guidelines should not be confused with empirical evidence supporting them (Pearson, Sabin & Emanuel, 1998; Berwick, 1996).

The framework involves asking a series of questions, each of which focuses on a dimension of the design of a capitation scheme. It also proposes "design principles" intended to answer these questions, at least in a general way. The first question asks what is at stake for a physician; that is, what is the magnitude or *intensity* of the incentives? The second asks how direct or *immediate* the risk is; that is, how many physicians share it for how many patients? A third asks, whether the incentives are *risk-adjusted* for the patient mix? Together, these three questions ask how strongly the physician feels the pressure of incentives to reduce utilization. The fourth question asks whether, how, and why incentives are *targeted* on specific services? The fifth pertains to how incentives are *balanced* between utilization reduction and quality improvement? These last two questions focus on how the incentives may affect standards of care.

There are several components to the intensity of the incentives. The *scope* of included services partly determines the intensity of risk. For example, if referrals for specialists or tests are included in the capitation, more frequent use of these services puts physicians at risk. The *amount* of money at stake—the potential dollars gained or lost in aggregate—also affects the intensity of incentives. Intuitively, for example, physicians will respond to incentives more—and will be perceived by patients to respond to them more—if the withholds or bonuses are 50% rather than 20% of the payment rate. The *structure* and *timing* of withholds and bonuses can create intense pressure at particular times, e.g., at the end of a year. Finally, since physicians may be particularly sensitive to actual losses, as opposed to foregone bonuses, the presence or absence of *stop-loss* provisions that limit the magnitude of financial loss physicians are exposed to significantly affect intensity.

The immediacy or directness of incentives depends on two factors: how many physicians and how many patients are involved. If incentives of a given intensity impose risks across a pool involving many physicians, a given physician making decisions about a particular patient will find them less intrusive than if there are fewer physicians sharing the risk. What each physician does has less impact on the aggregate result than if the risk is shared more narrowly. The same point holds for the numbers of patients.

If one physician has a sicker patient population than another, then, for a given intensity and immediacy of risk, the pressure imposed by incentives will be greater. Unfortunately, we have no developed method for risk-adjusting incentives to physicians, just as we have no adequate method for risk-adjusting reimbursements to health plans. Having noted the importance of this dimension, we set it aside in what follows.

What should physicians offer as evidence in order to justify the claim that the incentives they accept are "reasonable"? In the last section, we argued that patients and the public should recognize that some effort to motivate physicians to take population needs into account is reasonable. But what levels of intensity and immediacy are too great? When are patients justified in suspecting that their physicians are under too much pressure to violate the Primacy Principle?

The guidelines we are discussing propose as a design principle that systems not present an intensity of financial risk to individual physicians that "would lead reasonable persons to question whether physicians' judgments are improperly influenced." Similarly, they propose a design principle that capitation be used only for "large numbers of enrollees and only when there are methods available to diffuse financial risk or gain across a large number of providers." Unfortunately, the absence of appropriate, published empirical evidence about either physician behavior or patient perceptions makes it difficult to apply either design principle. When should reasonable persons question whether physician judgments are improperly influenced by the intensity of incentives? What is a large enough number of patients or providers?

In the absence of relevant empirical evidence about the actual behavior of physicians under incentives that vary in intensity and immediacy, physicians (and health plans) would have to adopt a conservative strategy. They would have to take patient and public skepticism seriously. They would have little evidence to show skeptical patients that might help demonstrate when intensity or immediacy is sufficient to prompt attention to limits without leading to violation of the Primacy Principle. Our point is that the task of persuading patients and the public that limits are reasonable requires openness, thought, and deliberation, and though the accountability for reasonableness framework is helpful in clarifying features of that deliberation, more empirical study is necessary to provide a basis for reasonable deliberation.

The remaining two questions, those concerning the targeting and balance of incentives, provide a good opportunity to evaluate how incentives affect the quality of care. Although patients primarily fear that incentives will cause harm by rewarding undertreatment (Kao, Zaslavsky, Green et al., 2001), incentives can be used to improve the standard of care. Showing that incentives are specifically aimed at improving care would go a long way toward demonstrating that patient-centered values form the core of efforts at limit setting.

Regarding targeting of specific services, the ethical guidelines propose that incentives should not "directly reward the decreased use of specific services unless: *1)* there is evidence of inappropriate utilization of those services; *2)* there are evidence-based methods for physicians to determine how to use the services more appropriately; and *3)* the services are monitored for underutilization." This design principle appropriately connects indirect limit setting to goals that fair-minded persons should admit are reasonable. Patients and the public have an interest in eliminating wasteful uses of services and in having evidence-based protocols guide clinical decisions. They also have an interest in quality assurance mechanisms that protect against underutilization.

Though these assurances that targeting is appropriately constrained by concerns about improving, or at least maintaining, quality of care, they still focus primarily on incentives aimed at reducing utilization. Incentives can, however, also reward physicians for specific behaviors that improve quality of care. For example, the incentives could reward physicians for achieving targets involving prevention, patient satisfaction, and clinical outcomes. Positive incentives to improve quality could go a long way toward counterbalancing fears of underutilization.

Perhaps a lesson can be drawn here from the design of the contract that exists between Massachusetts Behavioral Health Partnership, a for-profit company that contracts to deliver mental health services with the Massachusetts Division of Medical Assistance (see Chapter 9). Its contract specifies that a potential level of profit is achievable through the contract, but rather than the profits deriving primarily from lowering utilization, profits derive from meeting certain performance standards. This innovative contract achieves a reassuring balance since incentives aim to improve, for example, response times in emergency mental health care. The challenge facing designers of incentive systems for physicians is to develop a similar focus on quality improvement.

In sum, the framework of design principles we have discussed should better equip physicians and plans to answer the touchstone question, but their fundamental limitation—that they are based on theory and not empirical evidence about the effects of incentives—means they cannot completely answer the question. Health plans and physicians are in the difficult situation of not being able to demonstrate the reasonableness of their incentive systems without outcomes-based studies of their effects.

INSTITUTIONAL SUPPORT FOR PROFESSIONAL ETHICS

We have posed the touchstone question as one that physicians must answer: What are the arguments and evidence that should persuade *fair-minded* persons that an incentive scheme is a *reasonable* limit-setting device? To be publicly accountable for the reasonableness of incentive schemes, physicians should be comfortable with the evidence that those schemes pose no undue threat to the Primacy Principle and their patients' welfare. They should be no less equipped to explain the risks and benefits of these incentives to patients than they are to explain the risks and benefits of specific treatment options. In this way, public accountability for reasonableness supports a collaborative doctor–patient relationship.

Physicians cannot meet this challenge without institutional support. Health plans and negotiators for physician groups must have the touchstone question in mind when they bargain and plan or design incentive schemes, and employers should have them in mind when they contract with plans. They must ensure that it is a scheme for which an appropriate answer is possible, and this means they must support and perhaps sponsor research on the outcomes associated with incentives of various types. Existing arrangements provide excellent opportunities for the study of natural experiments (Rice & Gabel, 1996), but access to data and the ability to publish and share it are essential if accountability for reasonableness is to be possible. Ideally, standards, such those set by the National Committee on Quality Assurance (NCQA) could specify that incentives meet guidelines that are themselves based on evidence, and not just theory. We thus intend the device of the touchstone question to convert the process of establishing incentives into one in which there is evidence-based deliberation about the effects of incentives on patient welfare.

The task of persuading the public that reasonable limits to care, both direct and indirect, are part of a fair system involves education of physicians and health plan managers, as well as patients. The touchstone question, and more generally the task of holding plans and physicians accountable for the reasonableness of the limit setting they undertake, is intended to facilitate education over time. We are only at the beginning of a long learning curve since the problem of meeting diverse needs fairly under resource constraints is an unsolved problem of distributive justice that societies have just begun to address.

Changing a public culture so that the public understands and accepts reasonable limits to care and participates in establishing limits requires that we be explicit about rationales for the tool kits we use. It requires an explicit answer to the normative question: Should we trust physicians working with these incentives?

Our stand thus contrasts with reliance on more implicit means of managing trust, such as freeing physicians from the task of disclosing incentives at all. It also contrasts sharply with the reliance of current reform proposals on "rights to sue" health plans and "rights to rapid grievance procedures" in cases of denials (see Chapters 4 and 5). In the absence of reforms that change the culture of the health system into one where there is public accountability for the reasonableness of limits, such reforms perpetuate an adversarial, rather than collaborative, approach to setting limits to care, and they may even perpetuate the myth that patients can get whatever they want or need if they are litigious enough; that is, that the courts provide all the accountability that is needed.

Public accountability for reasonableness by physicians, plans, and agencies will also facilitate a broader public deliberation about the reasonableness of limits to health care. Ultimately, health plans and the medical profession, however entrepreneurial, must be accountable to democratic processes. But just as physicians and health plans are currently ill-equipped to deliberate thoughtfully about the reasonableness of indirect limits because they lack relevant evidence, so too is the public as a whole and its representatives in established political institutions. The careful effort of physicians and plans to answer the touchstone question and to be publicly accountable for doing so can engage the public in various ways, both direct and indirect, in the task of deliberation. This contribution is a necessary condition for establishing the legitimate moral authority of health plans to make limit-setting decisions—directly, as in coverage decisions, or indirectly, as in incentive schemes.

Our touchstone question is intended to highlight what physicians and health plans must do in order to preserve public confidence in professional ethics. Professional values require institutional support. They cannot simply be announced and avowed. Compliance with ethical principles, such as the Primacy Principle, requires not just individual commitment, but support of colleagues, the profession, other institutions, and the culture quite broadly. The design of incentive systems can be widely recognized either as a means of corrupting professional values or as a way to support them.

Our call for public accountability for reasonableness in the design and implementation of indirect methods of setting limits aims to support professional values by involving all these parties in deliberation about them.

NOTES

1. Massachusetts Medical Society Policy, Ethical Standards in Managed Care, (November 8, 1996); cf. American Medical Association, Council for Ethical and Judicial Affairs, Opinion 8.03 Conflicts of Interest (1998).

9

ACCOUNTABILITY FOR REASONABLENESS IN ACTION: PUBLIC SECTOR MENTAL HEALTH CONTRACTING

In the preceding chapters we have argued that accountability for reasonableness can help health plans and public agencies set limits that can be seen as legitimate and fair. We developed our initial ideas about fair process from studying how insurers and managed care organizations decide about coverage for new technologies. This area of decision-making has two distinctive features. It is episodic—programs must make yes or no decisions as new technologies emerge from their development phase. And, although we concluded that evidence alone does not eliminate the need for a fair process, extensive testing has generally been done, and reams of information are typically available. We decided to test our claim about the importance of accountability for reasonableness by applying it in a very different area—the use of private, for-profit, managed mental health care companies to provide public-sector mental health services. Public programs for citizens with severe mental illness are quintessential safety net services, provided within tight public budgets that require choices and trade-offs. In contrast to the domain of new technologies, decisions about priorities and limits in this area are ongoing, not episodic, and must often be made with much less information. We felt that, if accountability for reasonableness is not useful for managing this sector of public policy, there must be something wrong with the concept itself.

The public's nightmare image of for-profit, public-sector managed care is an impersonal, financially driven company siphoning public money away from needy citizens to line the pockets of greedy investors and lavishly paid executives. In a 1998 survey, twice as many adults enrolled in managed care than fee-for-service plans "worried that your health plan would be more concerned about saving money than about [providing] the best treatment for you if you are sick." While 72% of the sample agreed that managed care savings "helps health insurance companies to earn more profits," only 49% believed that that these savings also "makes health care more affordable for people like you" (Blendon, Brodie, Benson, et al., 1998).

Jokes capture public distrust of managed care even more vividly than the surveys: HMO means "Heave Mothers Out;" Utilization review means "1-800-Just-Say-No;" Saint Peter admits a surprised HMO medical director into heaven, "but only for two days—then, you will be discharged to the other place the way your HMO patients were."

Despite public attitudes towards managed care that range from skepticism to hatred, many states have hired for-profit managed mental health organizations to care for citizens with severe and persisting mental illnesses—one of the most difficult to treat populations. In the U.S. health care system, these patients have largely been excluded from private employer-based insurance. They have suffered from stigma and neglect. The public-sector safety net has generally provided whatever care they receive. The net is often porous, and many end up homeless or in jail. Most readers of this book will have encountered members of this population panhandling on the street or sitting in a doorstep with a bottle. Asking distrusted, for-profit managed care organizations to take responsibility for a hard-to-treat, stigmatized population sounds like a sick joke. How could it possibly be expected to work?

Medicaid is the most important source of funding for patients with severe and persisting mental illness. Medicaid programs are financed by a combination of federal and state funds but managed by the states, and, as of July 1998, 36 states were providing their Medicaid mental health services through managed care. Federal law governing Medicaid requires that services be "sufficient in amount, duration and scope to reasonably achieve their purpose" (Rosenbaum, Silver & Wehr, 1997, p. vii). The law, however, does not specify which "purposes" (e.g., clinical objectives) must be included. Traditional insurance contracts require "medically necessary" treatment, but the term "medical necessity" has no fixed meaning (Sabin & Daniels, 1994). As a result, public-sector clients, and the clinicians who serve them, must look to the contracting process between the state and the managed care organization to specify the expectations and values that will shape public-sector mental health goals.

With states moving from providing services to purchasing them, the quality of care and life for the vulnerable population we are concerned with in this chapter depends in large measure on the quality of the contracting process between the state and its managed care vendor. Contracts and the financing mechanisms they establish do not ensure quality. But as the premier authorities on the Medicaid contracting process state, they "influence conduct directly and indirectly and thus represent two of the health care system's most powerful drivers" (Rosenbaum, Silver & Wehr, 1997, p. vii). Since contracting is the central transaction between the purchaser and provider, we concluded that if accountability for reasonableness means anything anywhere, it would have to be here.

Providing needed treatment for patients with severe and persisting mental illness, while setting fair limits, is especially difficult because state-of-the-art treatment differs from treatment in other sectors of medicine. In addition to the familiar elements of health care—diagnostic evaluation, medication, hospitalization, and office-based counseling—effective treatment for this population also requires rehabilitation, housing, active outreach, and social support. A 1997 study in Wisconsin found that 40% of efficient state-of-the-art treatment for patients with serious and persisting mental illness, provided at a level of quality comparable to what health insurance typically covers for medical and surgical conditions, would not meet prevailing definitions of "medical necessity" (Hollingsworth & Sweeney, 1997). Advocates will press for more expansive coverage. Actuaries will guard the bottom line. Our theory suggested that accountability for reasonableness could help them come to mutually acceptable policies.

Among Medicaid managed mental health programs, Massachusetts and Iowa are widely regarded as flagship examples. Massachusetts is especially recognized for the way it uses performance standards in contracting (Sabin & Daniels, 1999a) and involves consumers and families in oversight of the managed care program (Sabin & Daniels, 1999b). Iowa is especially recognized for the way it diverts profits into community reinvestment (Sabin & Daniels, 2000b) and its constructive approach to defining "medical necessity" (Sabin & Daniels, 2000a). Therefore, in order to explore whether and how accountability for reasonableness could help public purchasers meet the needs of a chronically underserved, vulnerable population within a budget, we investigated how Massachusetts and Iowa sought to met this challenge in their Medicaid mental health programs. And, since Massachusetts and Iowa are both for-profit programs, we also used this study as an opportunity to see what perspectives accountability for reasonableness might provide on the controversial issue of for profit enterprise in health care.

Massachusetts.   Massachusetts has had the nation's first and largest statewide Medicaid managed mental health program, with approximately 450,000 recipients. Since 1995, its Medicaid mental health services have been provided by the Massachusetts Behavioral Health Partnership, a for-profit company owned by Value-Options, the largest provider of Medicaid behavioral health care carve-out services (3.7 million) and the second largest managed behavioral health care company

(20 million) (Mental Health Weekly, 1998, pp. 1, 4). (When an organization like Medicaid hires a specialty company like ValueOptions to provide mental health services, it is said to be "carving out" those services.)

The Massachusetts Division of Medical Assistance (Medicaid) espouses an activist philosophy of health care purchasing. According to former commissioner Bruce Bullen, "The prudent purchaser is not a passive buyer who merely selects the best value from among the choices offered [but one] who has a vision of what health care can—and should—be, and who . . . drives the marketplace towards objectives that the purchaser sets" (Bullen, 1998). To conduct this kind of activism, the purchaser must define quality and "express those definitions in purchasing specifications and work with contractors to meet them" (Bullen, 1998).

These are fine words and noble sentiments. But given public distrust of managed care, especially for-profit managed care, how can recipients of Medicaid-supported mental health services and the citizens of Massachusetts possibly trust a for-profit company to deliver the best possible care to the eligible population within the budget provided by the state? Won't the company inevitably stint on care delivery to improve its bottom line? Didn't Milton Friedman—the guru of capitalism—tell us that "there is one and only one social responsibility of business—to use its resources and engage in activities designed to increase its profits" (Friedman, 1970).

In the first negotiation between the Division of Medical Assistance and the Massachusetts Behavioral Health Partnership, the parties did indeed clash over the potential conflict between quality and profit. The state was concerned with ensuring high-quality care for Medicaid recipients at the lowest possible cost. The Massachusetts Behavioral Health Partnership wanted to provide high-quality care but wanted to make a reasonable profit at the same time. How could the state and the public trust the company if it earned more profit by spending less on care? How could the company accept a contract with too little potential for earnings? For a time, the parties were stymied. Then, they came up with an innovative idea.

Massachusetts recognized that its concern was with how much it got for its investment, not with the company's profits per se. It wanted a high-quality, efficient program that the public could trust. The state decided to tie profit potential to the achievement of performance targets, not to holding back on spending the budget allotted for clinical services. With each year of the contract, progressively more of the Massachusetts Behavioral Health Partnership's potential for profit has been attached to performance standards and less to achieving savings in service delivery. In 1996, 44% of the company's earning potential came from performance standards and 36% from savings in service delivery. In 1998, 67% came from meeting performance standards and only 20% from service savings.

The fact that the contract negotiation between the state and the Massachusetts Behavioral Health Partnership was conducted in accord with our Publicity and Relevance conditions fostered the development of the innovative agreement. Both parties were committed to an approach that would focus on the needs of individual patients and the larger population. Rewarding the managed care organization for not spending the service budget did not meet that requirement. Rewarding it for achieving clinically meaningful performance standards did. The performance-standard concept met the Relevance condition, and both parties felt comfortable bringing it into public discussion.

The 1997–1998 contract set 22 performance standards. Service users, the Alliance for the Mentally Ill, state officials from other departments, service providers, academic researchers, and other stakeholders participated in establishing the standards. Setting performance standards was a highly visible process, with extensive debate and participation. The standards focused on areas the stakeholders saw as important and needing improvement. Here are some examples:

- Patients who are discharged from the hospital with inadequate aftercare plans are susceptible to rapid readmission or even homelessness. The standard required that 95% of inpatient charts show that proper aftercare planning has been done.
- Sometimes hospitals do not involve the families or guardians of children and adolescents in treatment planning. Sometimes they try to do it, but the family or guardian is hard to contact. Whatever the cause, not involving families or guardians leads to worse outcomes. Because performance in this area had been worse than for adults, the standard was set lower—at 85%.
- Patients put onto medications in the hospital need to have those medications monitored when they leave. It is not uncommon for medication follow-up plans to break down. Without adequate follow-up, patients may experience avoidable medication complications or go off their medications altogether. A target of improving the previous year's performance by 7.5% was set for medication follow up within three weeks.

Performance standards are not the sole means through which the state defines its purchasing objectives. The body of the contract between the state and the Partnership creates numerous requirements. But performance standards provide a mechanism by which the state and the key Medicaid stakeholders can identify the areas they regard as especially important. A visitor to the offices of the Partnership sees the performance targets posted on nearly every wall. Interviews with major service providers in the Partnership's clinical network reveal that providers are well aware of the standards. The standards clearly represent an effort to use earning potential to transform "talk" about quality into the "walk" of performance. They give the purchaser, clients, families, providers of service, and the public the potential for choosing priorities the stakeholders regard as reasonable and holding the managed behavioral health care company accountable for achieving them. Performance standards provide a language that draws all stakeholders into deliberation about the goals of the program and focuses their disagreements on clinically relevant dimensions.

When we looked at how Massachusetts implemented the contract with the Massachusetts Behavioral Health Partnership, we saw that our initial concept of the Appeals Condition for accountability for reasonableness had to become more nuanced than a simple matter of legalistic appeals for policy exceptions. Contracting for reasonable services requires more than a preliminary negotiation, a document, a signature, and a mechanism for making appeals in the interim before a new contract. In Massachusetts, consumers, family members, providers, and the state are like highly involved parents, in constant interchange with the managed care program to steer the program in what they see as more reasonable directions. The process we saw was more like continuous quality improvement than legalistic appeal.

Consumers have two powerful direct channels of influence. The first is through a consumer advisory council, where consumers and advocates, joined by high-level representatives of Medicaid, the Department of Mental Health, and other key state agencies, meet monthly with staff from the managed care company. The council tries to focus on a small number of potentially high-leverage issues, such as clinical guidelines or the performance standards. We observed an extended discussion of a proposed guideline for treatment of depression. The group members critiqued the guideline on the basis of their own experience with medications. They commented that the guideline gave detailed advice about which medications to prescribe but said nothing about tailoring the regimen in ways that were acceptable to the patient. One member commented, "My therapist knows I won't take any medications before 6 p.m." They suggested that guidelines should discuss how the clinician can best collaborate with the patient in planning the treatment, commenting that this would make it likelier that the regimen will actually be followed. The final guideline incorporated the consumer recommendations.

Second, the Massachusetts Consumer Satisfaction Team initiative, an incorporated consumer-run project, assesses consumers' satisfaction with the services they receive. After extensive training, pairs of consumers and family members conduct a consumer-developed survey through face-to-face interviews with current service users. This initiative resulted from a combination of extended negotiations and planning among the Division of Medical Assistance (purchaser), the Massachusetts Behavioral Health Partnership (managed care organization), and consumer advocates. The survey findings go first to the provider organization and then to carve-out company staff responsible for managing the clinical network.

Several surveys disclosed that patients did not understand the rights they had under the state's patient rights legislation. The consumer-evaluators put questions about patient rights into the survey out of their own concern about making sure that patients were treated with respect. On the basis of the survey findings, several hospitals began to publicize the role of the human rights officer and to make that person more available to patients. Follow-up, six months later, showed that these improvements were continuing.

In addition, a statewide peer educators project provides a further avenue for consumer guidance regarding reasonable program performance. The peer project has trained 30 consumers to run recovery workshops, using a workbook developed for the purpose (Spaniol, Koehler, & Hutchinson, 1994). Peer-led sessions help persons with psychiatric disabilities understand the recovery process and develop practical skills. The leaders of the program are active members of the advisory councils and have extensive informal contact with the leadership of the managed care program. They use observations fed in by participants in the peer-led groups as a source of quality-relevant information. As an example, peer educators reported that Spanish-language services were deficient in a part of the state, which led to improvements in the program.

Families have structured access for influencing the Partnership through a family advisory council that functions similarly to the consumer advisory council. Family and foster-family representatives join with representatives of the state and the managed care company. Family members told us that, whatever the professional network provides, family members are often the most involved and knowledgeable "case managers" for a troubled child or adolescent. The family advisory council gave them a "direct opportunity to influence the movers and shakers of the system." When we asked about the council's most important accomplishment, they cited influencing two performance standards for 1999. First, they felt that many families did not understand how the complex treatment system worked. Through their advocacy, "develop(ing) and distribut(ing) printed resource materials for families/guardians intended to assist in maximizing youths' treatment experience" was adopted as a standard. Second, the group felt that a new program that provided adults with intensive coordination and planning services had been very successful (Sabin, 1998a). They succeeded in including a performance standard that required making those services available to children and adolescents as well.

Finally, providers meet regularly with the Partnership and the state as a professional advisory committee in the same kind of format as consumers and families. At one of the committee meetings, the group discussed outpatient utilization review, a common limit-setting mechanism through which managed care organizations review treatment plans for "appropriateness" and "medical necessity." Clinicians argued that the majority of treatment was relatively limited by agreement between clinician and patient. Why review treatments early when doing so wastes clinician time and company resources for little benefit with regard to establishing reasonable limits? The company agreed and instituted an automated approval system clinicians could use via a simple touch-telephone procedure.

The Massachusetts program has built the essence of accountability for reasonableness into the annual goal-setting process and its ongoing monitoring. In setting performance standards, the state listens carefully to recommendations from consumers, families, and the clinical community as to what the top priorities should be. The same parties participate in regular monitoring of progress with regard to the standards and in the annual cycle of setting new ones.

Iowa.   Iowa is a rural state seven times larger than Massachusetts but with only half the population. As of 1990, 79 of Iowa's 99 counties had populations under 30,000. A 1996 survey showed that almost half of the 211 psychiatrists in the state practiced in one of three counties. Two-thirds of the counties have no psychiatrist. Iowa has four state mental health institutions, one in each of the four geographic quadrants of the state. Prior to the advent of managed care, the mental health system was highly decentralized with substantial county control. This close-knit rural state has been the unlikely site of an illuminating drama involving a turbulent collision between late 20th century capitalism and the public-sector values of safety net and asylum. Out of this collision, and the public deliberation it engendered, Iowa developed an innovative way of dealing with profit itself.

Iowa began to use managed care for its Medicaid medical/surgical program in 1986. That experience was largely positive, and, in 1993, the governor asked the Department of Human Services to create a statewide managed mental health program. After receiving the needed federal Medicaid approvals, the Department issued a request for proposals (RFP) for what was first called the Mental Health Access Plan (MHAP) in March of 1994. Eight companies submitted proposals. When the contract was awarded to Value Behavioral Health (now ValueOptions), Medco (subsequently Merit Behavioral Care, now part of Magellan), which ranked second, sued on the grounds that the Department of Human Service's consultant (Lewin-VHI) and Value Behavioral Health were both owned by the same parent company.

The court agreed that, despite the state's efforts to insulate the procurement process from the consultation, "as a sister subsidiary of Value, Lewin-VHI had motive and opportunity to share inside information with Value that was not available to other bidders." In July 1994, the Iowa Supreme Court upheld the original ruling, stating that the case "involved an organizational conflict of interest that was incapable of mitigation" (Rohland, 1996). In November 1994, the state, which had elected not to appeal, awarded the contract to Medco/Merit Behavioral Care of Iowa. Merit began covering patients under the Mental Health Access Plan on March 1, 1995.

Starting a contract with a lawsuit is like starting a marriage in a divorce court— not an auspicious launch for what needs to be a collaborative process—and the conflict and turmoil that landed the bidding process in court did not end with the signing of the contract. Both Merit staff and state officials described the first year of the program as "very rocky." One state official reported that in the first six months, "we came close to pulling the plug." Part of the problem was operational, especially slow claims payment. But the central source of turmoil was a clash between the way medical necessity criteria are used to set limits in the private sector and the requirements of public sector safety net functions.

Managed mental health care in the United States cut its teeth and achieved its early cost-containment success in the private sector in the late 1980s and early 1990s. Some of the initial results were relatively easy to achieve. Hospitals were often used when a less intensive form of care could achieve the same or even better results. To a large degree, private sector managed mental health care earned its initial spurs by cultivating skill at saying no.

Private-sector contracts typically define "medical necessity" in terms of symptom remission and return to baseline functioning. This definition is adequate for meeting the needs of a well-functioning person with reliable environmental supports who experiences an acute illness. It is not reasonable, however, for many persons in the public sector whose severe mental illness has caused progressive deviation from the potential they might have achieved without the impact of the illness and who may live in circumstances of socioeconomic deprivation.

The state and its vendor treated the initial eruption over how to define "medical necessity" as if it were an emergency appeal process. Where other public contracts have self-destructed in similar situations, Iowa and Merit were able to use the conflict as an opportunity for deliberation and quality improvement. Out of this process the state and the vendor identified three specific ways in which private sector medical necessity limits were not reasonable when applied to a public program.

Initially, Merit balked at covering court-ordered inpatient evaluations when the clinical situation did not meet their "necessity" criteria for hospital care. Court-ordered evaluations, however, are often last-resort safety net functions for high-visibility, high-concern situations, in which the court sends an alleged offender who seems mentally abnormal to a hospital for evaluation. It is one thing to conclude that a private-sector patient no longer needs acute hospital care and can be discharged home. It is quite different to discharge a possible felon whom the court has sent to the hospital for clinical assessment. Merit changed the policy to cover up to five days for court-ordered inpatient evaluation, or one day for substance abuse evaluation, regardless of their assessment of whether the enrollee's condition required hospital care for strictly clinical reasons.

Second, Iowa, like many other states, has had great difficulty creating enough residential settings for disturbed children and adolescents who cannot remain at home but who do not require acute hospital level care. In the initial implementation phase, children and adolescents who no longer met medical necessity criteria for inpatient care were sometimes discharged before a satisfactory alternative became available. Here, too, the conflict led to a change of policy and practice. Under a new "Keep Kids Safe" policy, children and adolescents are not discharged from inpatient care until a safe living arrangement was available and a plan for the necessary follow-up mental health treatment had been arranged. In the first year after this change, 194 children were kept in the hospital for an average of 17.6 days more than purely clinical needs required. Keeping troubled children in the hospital does not solve the societal problem of inadequate residential sites, but it avoids making the problem worse by discharging children who do not have a proper site to receive them.

Finally, Merit and the state shifted from the hard-nosed private-sector concept of medical necessity to a new combination of "medical" and "psychosocial" necessity that sets limits in a way that is better attuned to public-sector responsibilities. Merit and the state agreed to define "psychosocial necessity" as "an expansion of medical necessity" that examines "environmental factors that inhibit or hamper the effectiveness of [treatment] unless they are addressed" (Merit Behavioral Care of Iowa, 1996a, p. 6). "Psychosocial necessity" includes rehabilitative and supportive services as well as traditional clinical services, and the frontline managed care staff are told to consider "the potential for services/supports to allow the enrollee to maintain functioning improvement attained through previous treatment" (Merit Behavioral Care of Iowa, 1996b, p.23). It leads to limits seen as more reasonable in the public-sector context.

Like Massachusetts, Iowa's experience in contracting for mental health services touched on the fundamental question of what the public could accept as a reasonable approach to profit for the managed care company. In the initial contract, 81% of the capitation was for paying claims and 19% for administrative costs. The contract specified that any savings from the claims fund would be divided between the state and the carve-out vendor, with 80% going to the state and 20% to Merit. However, when it became apparent that there would be unspent monies in the claims fund, something interesting and unexpected happened. The state and the managed care company found themselves feeling "embarrassed" at the prospect of earning profit (for the company) or surplus (for the state) from public resources that had been earmarked for care and could otherwise be used to provide benefit for Iowa citizens (Surles, 1997). The embarrassment was a direct result of the Publicity Condition, as the fact of the savings and the way the initial contract would have distributed them would be in the public domain.

Experienced clinicians monitor and use subjective experience as data for guiding the treatment process. Experienced administrators use subjective experience in much the same way with regard to the management process. The state and its vendor interpreted the embarrassment they felt about the use of unspent treatment funds as an indicator that the original contract was not reasonable and should be modified. They were wise enough to recognize that, like a formal appeal, "embarrassment" provided data about the system and should trigger a learning process.

The state and the vendor concluded that, even if the funds were not needed for acute care within the network as it existed, the network itself could be improved. This is what made taking the unspent funds as surplus or profit feel embarrassing. This realization led them to revise the contract. For 1996 and 1997, the state and Merit agreed to reinvest approximately $1 million per year of what would otherwise have been surplus or profit into strengthening the service system. The program was well received, and the new contract that took effect on January 1, 1999, incorporated several innovations based on the experience of the first contract.

In the new contract, 83.5% of the $58 million Medicaid contract goes into claims, 2.5% into community reinvestment, and 14% to the company for administration. The contract provides that, if any money remains in the claims fund at the end of the year, it will go towards community reinvestment. The company's opportunities for profit beyond what is contained in the administrative component come from performance indicators. Eight performance indicators have incentive payments of $125 thousand attached to them, creating the potential of an additional $1 million in profit for meeting the performance targets. Ten performance indicators carry penalties only, to be paid into the community reinvestment fund if the standards are not met. The absence of controversy in the highly public contracting process suggests that Iowa citizens and advocates regard this new approach to profit as reasonable.

Like the performance standards in Massachusetts, the community reinvestment program provides an arena for deliberation among stakeholders about how the Iowa system can best be improved. The only way to reduce expenditure on costly hospital-level services is to strengthen community resources. The community reinvestment program provides one-year grants that allow providers to invest in community-based programs which, if successful, can be funded on a fee-for-service basis thereafter. Here are two examples:

- A grant to the Gannon Center in Dubuque allowed the Center to hire staff for a drop-in and crisis intervention program. Under the grant, the program ran for 40 hours a week, which was reduced to 20 hours a week when the grant ended. By consumer preference, the program operates primarily on weekends when there is little social opportunity in the downtown area where many of the consumers live.

  If outpatient services must be precertified for payment, a flexible drop in program is stymied by not being able to specify in advance when its clients will actually drop in! Merit Behavioral Care of Iowa and the Gannon Center worked out a system whereby the managed care program precertifies a specified number of visits for a three-month period for each client. If fewer visits are used, the full number is not billed for. If more are used, they are generally covered. The company allows the Gannon Center to backdate a certification form for visits that have not been anticipated.

- Several community reinvestment grants went to peer-support programs. Not all of these succeeded, but the pilot experience allowed the managed care program to create a set of specifications under which it would pay fee-for-service for peer support. Thus when Hope Haven in Rock Valley, in a sparsely populated rural area of northwest Iowa, developed a plan for peer-support services, it was able to establish them as billable. Hope Haven hires, trains, and supervises consumer peer support specialists, who provide outreach services that are authorized and paid for through the standard process. The executive director reports that "we can sit down with the people who are funding the service to solve problems—the care managers act like partners."

CONCLUSION

The ultimate way for Massachusetts and Iowa to be accountable for the reasonableness of their mental health policies would be to demonstrate the positive impacts of their programs on the health of the insured populations, but, like the other 48 states, they have relatively skimpy outcome data. The contracting process between the two states and the managed mental health companies, however, still has much to teach about how to use contracting a vehicle for defining reasonable targets, holding the insurer accountable for the reasonableness of its performance, and setting limits in a way that can be seen as legitimate and fair. The contract and its implementation move accountability for reasonableness into the realm of a contractual expectation, fulfilling the fourth condition—public regulation.

At the most basic level, citizens of both states share the national concern about allowing health organizations, especially for-profit organizations, to earn more by doing less—by not spending funds potentially available for care. Massachusetts built the principle of tying financial incentives to clinically meaningful performance standards into its contract. In Iowa, the first contract was structured so that the state and the company profited by not spending the claims fund, but the parties were wise enough to recognize that the "embarrassment" they felt at doing what the contract allowed meant that something in the contract was not reasonable. That recognition led them to preclude making a profit by not spending funds that had been earmarked for treatment and to the idea of community reinvestment. The expectation that policies would be shared with the public and that they would be based on reasons relevant to improving the health of individuals and the population led to innovative ways of tying a profit motive to the health goals of the two state programs.

It is hard to picture a private-sector purchaser and managed care program voluntarily reducing their contractually allowed potential for profit or surplus as occurred in Iowa. There is no reason to believe that public-sector employees are inherently more charitable than those in the private sector. Public-sector programs are, however, subjected to scrutiny by concerned stakeholders in ways that private programs are not. Because they are embedded in an open political process they have wider accountabilities than private-sector programs do. This wider accountability fostered a collaborative learning and quality improvement process that has thus far served Iowa well.

Massachusetts enhances the potential for establishing policies that embody acceptable limits by creating opportunity for meaningful consumer, family, and provider voice at key leverage points in the policy development process. By involving key stakeholders in setting performance objectives, defining clinical guidelines, and evaluating quality, the state gives recurrent opportunity for shaping policies that address the priorities of both individuals and the population and whose rationales are publicly understood.

Public entities like state governments and the Medicaid program are required by statute to meet the Publicity Condition of accountability for reasonableness, so it is not surprising to find innovative approaches to accountability in exemplary public programs. The specific practices, however, could be transferred to the private sector as well. If it hopes to address the vehement public backlash against it, private-sector managed care will have to guide itself by public-sector practices like those in Iowa and Massachusetts.

10

AN INTERNATIONAL LEARNING CURVE

As we said in the first sentence of the first chapter, all societies face a common problem: how to meet health care needs fairly under resource constraints. Thus far, our examples of limit setting are taken largely from the United States. In this chapter, we look at a series of examples from other countries with important differences from the United States. Denmark, the Netherlands, New Zealand, Norway, and Sweden (Sections 2 and 3) all asked public commissions to provide an explicit framework for limit setting and rationing in a way that has not occurred in the United States, with the notable exception of Oregon. Unlike these countries but like the United States, Britain (Section 4) has relied on implicit limit-setting processes with no national commission to deal with rationing, but, unlike the United States, the British have universal access and a national budget. Developing countries, exemplified by Colombia, Mexico, Pakistan, and Thailand (Section 5) address limits within systems that have many fewer resources.

Despite substantial differences in design, financing, political culture, and resources, all of these countries are part of a broad learning curve for dealing with a common problem. Taking this global perspective allows a series of conclusions (Section 6) about what we humans have learned about fair health care limit setting as of the turn of the millennium. Accountability for the reasonableness of limit-setting decisions emerges as a necessary condition for establishing and sustaining the legitimacy of these decisions in all systems.

CONTRASTING PUBLIC MESSAGES

On the face of it, how countries like Norway or Denmark, or the Netherlands or Canada, face the problem of resource scarcity and limits to care would seem to have nothing to do with what will happen or what must be done in the United States. To Americans, including policy makers, their differences from us seem to overwhelm any similarities. The American public is rarely directed to look abroad for lessons we might learn. Indeed, during periods when universal coverage has been on the American policy agenda, Americans have often been barraged by a campaign of disinformation aimed at spreading as much skepticism as possible about national health insurance systems.

The differences between American and other developed country systems are, of course, significant. Other advanced industrialized countries have universal coverage. The United States, alone among them, does not. As a result, some 45 million Americans, or 11 times the population of Norway, are without insurance. All of these systems, despite their financing and organizational variations, promise a comprehensive set of benefits to their whole populations. Most of them include all, or nearly all, health care costs within global national budgets. In some of them, such as the Nordic countries, all hospitals are publicly owned. Funding is either from general tax revenues or from compulsory contributions based on income but is unrelated to illness or use of the system. In contrast, the U.S. system has multiple financing streams, varied levels of benefits for different population subgroups, extensive private control over levels of coverage, and no global budget.

Because of the design of their health care institutions, people in these systems share a common experience. For them, problems facing the system become shared problems requiring shared solutions. By design, the system makes it clear to the public that everyone is in it together. The moral and political commitment to solidarity that contributes to people accepting universal coverage in the first place is in turn reinforced by the benefits all derive from it. Just as culture influences institutions, so too institutions influence political culture.

In the United States, people do not identify with "our" system in the same way, in part because their experience of the system varies so much from group to group. Some have insurance; some don't. Some are on Medicaid; most have insurance through their employers. Some are on Medicare; most are not, although all who live long enough eventually will be (which helps explain the strong support for this system). Around half of those ensured by their employers have some choice among health plans, but the rest do not. Problems people experience with their health plans, such as denials of coverage for treatment, may seem isolated to the health plan their employer has chosen for them or the one they may have chosen themselves. They may even see it as their own mistake—they purchased the wrong plan.

In general, when Americans encounter limits to care or other problems in medical delivery, they are more likely to think of them as the result of a "bad" plan, or bad behavior by a particular plan or individuals. In the backlash to managed care, the print and electronic media have linked the diverse experiences of patients and physicians and focused the blame for restrictions on a common source. As a result, many people increasingly believe that the problem is caused by managed care and the expansion of for-profit health care.

Americans, however, do not see the problem as a manifestation of resource scarcity and the (perhaps inappropriate) management of necessary limits. We cannot see it as a collective problem that transcends managed care because everything in our experience and in the public messages we hear tells us it is not. To Americans, the message that costs are rising too rapidly does not translate in the public mind into the understanding that resources are limited (as we noted in Chapter 1). Instead, it translates into other messages: employers do not want to pay enough; taxes are too high; or companies are seeking to raise profits.

In contrast to the American perception, in the mid- to late 1980s, awareness began to grow in many universal coverage systems that there was a national problem of resource limits that called for making choices about what kind of care to provide. Complaints about growing waiting lists and inquiries and demands about new kinds of services made it clear that public awareness of existing limits had grown and had to be addressed. The problem was talked about in varying terms—"setting limits," "establishing priorities," "making choices"—but it was generally seen as collectively affecting shared public, or publicly managed, resources. Not surprisingly, shared problems demanded agreement on fair solutions, and a wave of national commissions—in Norway (Norges Offentliche Utredninger, 1987), the Netherlands (Ministry of Welfare, Health and Cultural Affairs, 1992), Denmark (Danish Council of Ethics, 1996), Finland (National Research and Development Centre, 1995), Sweden (Sveriges Offentliga Utredningar, 1995), and elsewhere—reported on their deliberations about choices, priorities, and limits (Holm, 2000).

In the United States, there have been no comparable national commissions to discuss limits, choices, or priorities. There is no public acknowledgment of a problem of scarcity and priorities. Of course, there is a problem—sometimes portrayed as a crisis—of increasing costs. Rising costs, however, are primarily seen as the result of inefficiency and waste or as the result of excessive demand by patients and physicians who "feel no price." Inefficiency, so the argument goes, is a problem for market solutions, not bureaucratic regulation.

In the United States, political leaders, health policy experts, and the health industry have all sent the same message: rely on the market to control costs, change reimbursement incentives from fee for service to capitated arrangements, and establish competition among plans, and costs will be controlled. As we noted in Chapter 1, when national health insurance was on the agenda, the problem of setting limits or rationing was ruled out of bounds—not to be discussed at all—so confident were the managers of the Clinton Health Care Task Force that competition would eliminate waste and inefficiency and, thus, all need to talk about resource limits.

The sole exception to the official policy line in the United States was Oregon's effort to set priorities within Medicaid. Although the Oregon plan found little support elsewhere in the country, it was greeted warmly by Europeans as an intriguing initiative to involve the public in deliberation about priorities and limits.

Still, what distinguished Oregon's effort from European concerns may have been more important than what they shared. Unlike European programs, Oregon's was not really aimed at "our" system, one shared by all the public. In Oregon, the prioritization plan was for "their" Medicaid system, insurance for the poor. Despite the solid democratic intentions of many involved in the Oregon effort, and the fact that its proponents hoped to expand it to cover a broad segment of the population, the plan could not avoid the appearance of the "haves" setting priorities for the "have-nots" (Daniels, 1991). To most Americans, the response to Oregon (where there was awareness of it) would most likely have been, "Of course, resources for the poor are limited, but that has nothing to do with 'our' health care." Thus, despite Oregon, Americans have not acknowledged or publicly addressed the problem that has been stage center on the agenda of universal coverage systems.

As Americans begin the 21st century, public discussion of major reform of the health system has receded. There is neither discussion of universal coverage nor of limit setting. Instead, policy discussion focuses on improving quality in the system. In part, this is a reaction to the anxiety produced by cost-reduction efforts of the last decade, but it is also stimulated by Institute of Medicine reports of threats to patient safety and quality of care. In this context, broad public discussion of limit setting is again made less likely.

INITIAL EUROPEAN EFFORTS: THE SEARCH
FOR SIMPLE SOLUTIONS

The national commissions established by Norway, Denmark, the Netherlands, Sweden, and other countries to discuss health care priorities or choices mark an important first point on a social learning curve. In all of these commission reports, there is a discussion of the importance of eliminating waste and inefficiency, and many of these systems have introduced market-mimicking mechanisms, often adapted from U.S. models, to address these problems. The main point, however, of these commissions is the need to recognize and address a deeper problem.

The deeper problem of limits is analyzed in all these reports as the result of several health policy successes, not failure. First, various public health and other measures have succeeded in changing the disease profile in advanced industrialized societies, replacing acute infectious diseases with chronic diseases as the major sources of morbidity and mortality. Second, the shift has helped to cause, and is in turn partly caused by, the aging of our populations. Third, investments in medical technologies have produced treatments that are effective ways to improve quality of life, even for those with chronic disease. The more we know about the potential of these new treatments, the more we demand them—even if many of them make modest improvements at considerable cost. Since, however, health care is not the only social good, and other social goals must also be pursued, we have to set limits to health care by establishing priorities and making choices.

The first wave of national commissions not only analyzed the problem, promoting public understanding of it, but argued in favor of various principles and methods for establishing priorities (Holm, 2000). The influential 1987 Norwegian report urged that priorities be set by ranking initiatives or interventions into one of five levels depending on the seriousness of the disease or condition addressed. The 1994 Finnish report and the 1995 Swedish Parliamentary Priorities Commission Report were both modeled on the Norwegian approach.

In the Norwegian scheme, highest priority would be given to interventions that were necessary because of imminent risk to the lives of individuals or groups. For example, emergency medicine, including the treatment of acute infectious diseases, was paradigmatic here. The second tier involved interventions needed to address diseases with catastrophic, but not imminent, consequences for individuals or groups. Third were interventions whose applicability was documented but where the consequences were not as serious as in the first two categories, as in the treatment of moderately high blood pressure or moderate psychological problems. The fourth level involved initiatives that improved health and quality of life, but where the consequences of non-treatment were less significant. Some reproductive and infertility services were included here. Services that were neither necessary nor of unambiguously documented applicability were given lowest priority. The Swedish model invoked a similar ranking, but it distinguished between priority setting at the political or administrative levels and at the clinical level.

A key moral belief behind the Norwegian scheme was that we must give priority to those with the most serious conditions. A central problem was that the model provided no way to take into account the degree of effectiveness of treatments or their costs. Many who accept the importance of giving priority to those whose conditions make them worst off would still want to balance that priority against our ability to improve their conditions through effective interventions. Many would further argue that we should balance even effective measures aimed at the worst-off patients against their "opportunity cost," that is, the benefits we forgo for others. Thus, producing marginal gains for the worst off, but at very high cost, may involve forgoing morally more important benefits to others. The very simplicity of the scheme meant it ignored some of the complexity of the moral problem it addressed.

Soren Holm (2000), a former member of the Danish Ethics Council on whose work we draw in this and the next section, argues that the variations on this scheme, adopted in the Nordic countries, embodied an early hope that decision rules could be formulated for priority setting that would work simply and eliminate controversy. He notes that even if some measure of effectiveness and cost had been introduced, as in cost effectiveness analysis, the same goal of explicit, simple rules (and simple tools) would have dominated the approach. In support of his view, it is worth noting that Oregon, working in this same early period of public discussion, had initially adopted an approach that incorporated measures of effectiveness and cost. Its avowal of cost-effectiveness ranking reflected the same goal of providing a clear way of establishing priorities among all services. The ranking was to be driven by "the facts"—the numbers about costs and medical benefits. The actual rationing in Oregon would then be left to the legislature, which, aware of the consequences of different levels of funding, would make a public choice about what benefits to exclude. As we noted earlier, the simplicity of Oregon's cost-effectiveness approach led it to violate the point—giving special priority to the worst off—behind the Norwegian ranking. Oregon, in the face of public protest against the results of a priority-setting process that depended on the single factor of cost-effectiveness, adopted a more complex approach to ranking services (Hadorn, 1991).

The 1992 Dutch report on Choices in Health Care, which Holm includes in his "first phase" of "simple solutions," argued for a set of four criteria to guide all legislative decisions about the contents of the basic health care package. Specifically, these four criteria were depicted as a series of filters through which all services passed in order to be funneled into the universal basic benefit package: *a)* is it necessary care, from the community point of view? *b)* is it demonstrated to be effective? *c)* is it efficient? *d)* can it be left to individual responsibility? The committee illustrated its reasoning from these criteria, arguing, for example, that in vitro fertilization was not necessary from a community perspective, even though individuals might feel it was necessary from an individual one. The committee also used the same criteria to argue that sports injuries, even if they resulted from lifestyle choices individuals made, should not be excluded from the basic benefit package, because there was uncertainty about whether such exclusions would have a net positive or negative effect on population health.

Neither the simple Norwegian scheme nor the more complex Dutch one avoided controversy. The Norwegian scheme, however simple the decision rules seem, encouraged lobbying about what diseases or conditions should be placed in the various priority categories. Getting one's disease viewed as more serious meant getting higher priority in resources.

Disagreements about priority often rest on the complexity of the notion of the seriousness of a condition. Analyzing the seriousness of a condition or disease into its several components requires distinguishing "urgency" (how quickly the disease will have its effect without treatment) from "functional impact" (how extensively the disease impacts on functioning or life expectancy whenever its effect is felt).

Obviously, there will be trade-offs between urgency and functional impact, and deciding how to make these will bring disagreements. For example, depending on how much weight people give to urgency as compared to impact, they might not rank everything in the second category below items in the first.

The Dutch scheme, given its own examples, also invited considerable disagreement and controversy. Is infertility really only an individual and not a community problem? When it came to implementing the system, public pressure altered the priority given to infertility treatments—there was a clear political response to the power of advocacy groups. In effect, the simple rules were not so simple to apply, and the decisions that were allegedly made on the basis of them could still be contested as arbitrary and unfounded.

In Denmark, according to the Danish Council of Ethics Report on Priority Setting (1996), different counties modified and applied versions of the Norwegian scheme in somewhat different ways. The County of Sorstrom, for example, developed a seven-category scheme. It was greeted with "turbulent and heated debate" when it became clearer what the implications were for the treatment of specific conditions (Danish Council, 1996, p. 63). Further, not all patients seemed to fit neatly into the seven categories, and the ways in which seriousness of condition and effectiveness of treatment conflicted became apparent.

The difficulties that emerged when these early schemes for setting priorities were implemented reflect points we made in earlier chapters. We argued that general principles of distributive justice were indeterminate with regard to key unsolved rationing problems, leaving considerable room for reasonable disagreement. That inability to guide actual rationing decisions meant that fair process must supplement appeals to general principles. The difficulties faced by these early efforts are examples of this underlying problem. The attempts to reconcile concerns about seriousness of need and effectiveness of treatment, to say nothing of costs and efficiency, already involved reasonable disagreements about how to interpret and apply these concepts to specific cases. Consequently, commission articulation of general principles and goals of the system did not resolve reasonable disagreements, since principles and goals conflicted.

Before describing a second phase of Nordic responses to the problem—a further point on the social learning curve in some countries—it is worth noting that not all universal coverage systems, including those in which there is public ownership of most hospitals and funding through general tax revenues, have addressed the problem through an open discussion by a national commission. In Great Britain, for example, there have been extensive discussions by academics and others about how resources in the National Health Service (NHS) should be allocated, and the King's Fund and others have focused public attention on the need for more thought about rationing. But the main focus of public discussion has been on how measures to improve efficiency would protect the ability of the system to continue to provide all beneficial services, and there has been considerable government re-sistance to opening or leading a discussion of rationing. We return later to further discussion of some lessons from the more recent British experience, including its introduction of a central mechanism for technology assessment.

A SECOND WAVE OF EUROPEAN EFFORTS: A FOCUS ON FAIR PROCESS

The Danish Council of Ethics 1996 report *Priority-setting in the Health Service,* marked an effort to move beyond the simple solutions criticized by Holm (2000). So did a second Norwegian national report issued in 1997. Neither report denied the value of attempting to articulate criteria and to have a public debate about them. Both reaffirmed the importance of doing that. The Danish report, for ex-ample, engaged in a detailed discussion of which criteria were appropriate and in-appropriate at both political and clinical levels of priority setting (adopting the Swedish distinction about levels of priority setting).

Nevertheless, the Danish report emphasized the fact that articulating criteria for priority setting and attempting to use them in actual settings must be seen as fram-ing a public debate, not resolving it. Holm (2000), commenting on the Danish Council report, remarks that early national reports oversimplified the problem, at-tempting to focus too narrowly on one purpose among several of a health care sys-tem. A health care system does not merely treat disease, or meet health care needs, or ensure equality in health. It also heightens security and publicly reflects concerns about solidarity. How these goals should be balanced in actual priority setting is not captured by overly simple schema. In practice, the schema for set-ting priorities actually gave little real guidance to decision makers. Even where the schema were used to set priorities, for example, to specify waiting time guaran-tees based on severity categories, doctors "gamed" the system to gain advantage for their own patients—and room for their gaming was provided by the many ways in which severity could be reinterpreted. Not only did clinicians undermine the priorities to serve their own patients, but, in some highly publicized cases, politicians undercut the appeal to them in response to constituent demands.

Turning their attention away from simple priority schemes, both the Danish and Norwegian reports focused on the importance of fair process in the actual setting of priorities. In striking language, the Danish Report (p. 95) emphasized trans-parency and the importance of debate and dialogue:

> The Danish Council of Ethics is of the opinion that in planning the operation of the health service, and not least in connection with priority-setting in the health service, *openness and dialogue* concerning the decisions made should be ensured. This open-ness is to be inward as well as outward. There should be an effort to ensure that

decision-makers at different levels become aware—informed—of which priority-setting consequences different decisions entail. . . . At the same time the public should also be ensured a higher level of information on which decisions are made at which levels, and which reasons there are for individual decisions. Such openness is crucial to ensuring that individual decisions can be subjected to criticism and possibly changed on the basis of the public debate. For this reason great importance should also be attached to the health planning in counties being organized in such a way as to ensure the possibility for common citizens to participate in the decision-making process, for instance at hearings and public meetings.

As if to take up the Danish report's challenge, the Norwegian Report of 1997 (Norges Offentlige Utredninger, 1997; referred to as Lonning II) goes even further in specifying elements of fair process, for example, in the development of clinical guidelines that can help establish the legitimacy of the limits they impose. The deliberation is initially carried out by specialty-specific groups, but these groups must show what such general criteria as severity, utility, and efficiency mean in the context of their work. They must then recommend priorities based on that analysis. Decisions about these priorities are ultimately to be made at a political level, but the political process is informed by the deliberation of the specialty groups. The goal is to make decisions about limits accountable to those affected by them and to be clear that the grounds for those limits are rooted in a grasp of the evidence regarding treatments and their importance to patients and population health.

In discussing the implementation of the 1997 Norwegian report, Norheim (Norheim, Ekeberg, Evens, et al., 2001) notes that clinical guidelines also function as a rationing tool. For example, one of the criteria that applies in developing a guideline is the importance of the guideline, that is, "whether it can reduce local variation in practice, have an impact on management, or have an impact on major outcomes or costs" (Norheim, 2000 p. 5). But the distribution of this impact is also important, and the consequences must be acceptable to patients. To accomplish this end, Norheim argues, this group of stakeholders must be involved in guideline development. Real transparency would mean unpacking the value components that are often disguised as clinical judgments—in this case, of the importance of the guideline. Ensuring that those value components are acceptable to those affected by the decisions requires, Norheim suggests, some form of public participation in guideline development.

Norheim also notes that there are obstacles to making rationales for limits accessible to patients in the context of physicians complying with guidelines. Most important, there are no incentives to the physician to provide for the transparency and explicitness needed for patients to engage with the reasons for these limits and to accept them—or to have a clear basis for challenging them. Whether it was because of these obstacles or for other reasons, few recommendations of the Lonning II commission were implemented as of 2001 (Norheim, 2001).

Altogether, Norheim provides a sobering assessment of the degree to which

Norwegian reforms captured the key elements of accountability for reasonableness. First, though there was a call for transparency in the development of guidelines and in the introduction of an appeals process for cases of denials of treatment for services abroad, there was inadequate public accessibility. Where guidelines for new bone marrow transplant technologies were promulgated, they were publicly available, but not in a form that made them publicly understandable. The government appeals board provided inadequate access to public inquiries about its decisions. Similar problems faced compliance with the Relevance Condition: because it was difficult to understand the reasons for policies, it was also difficult to judge whether the reasons were relevant. In contrast to many other universal coverage systems, the Norwegians have at least two forms of appeal boards for denials of care—for treatment abroad and for appeals from clinical guidelines. The guideline appeals, however, are only advisory and not formal decision-making procedures. What emerges, then, is the fact that despite public discussion and a history of commissions grappling with the need to implement fair process, implementation is piecemeal and uneven.

Norheim's (2001) critical discussion of implementation of elements of the process required by Lonning II shows that there is a remarkable convergence with the central ideas of accountability for reasonableness, even as continued learning about the features of fair process is underway and as implementation is slow and uneven. Though the route to this focus began in the Nordic countries with national commissions leading a public discussion of priority setting, there is no one path to discovering the importance of such accountability. We illustrate some other paths in the following sections.

The Nordic countries are not alone in following this evolution in their approach to rationing. New Zealand shows a similar trend (Edgar, 2000). Following health reform efforts in 1991 that many saw as a threat to the social contract around health care, a significant effort at public involvement and education about limits to care was undertaken. A series of public reports on rationing were issued, all of which involved public participation. The first, *Best of Health* (NHC, 1992), raised publicly the need for setting limits and posed issues about what kinds of trade-offs in services might be involved. As this document was discussed in town hall meetings and through questionnaires, public opinion concerning priorities among service categories was gathered. The process here had some similarities to Oregon's efforts to clarify public values in its rationing program. Public concerns—for example, that basic services be available closer to home and that community care was preferred to institutional care—influenced later purchasing initiatives.

In 1993, *The Best of Health 2* (NHC 1993) asked the public how decisions should be made about publicly funded services. In the discussion that followed, there was considerable support for a framework that included consideration of benefit, value for money, fairness in access and resource use, and consistency with other community values. In addition to these large-scale efforts to obtain public opinion, there were many consensus conferences among experts on specific issues, such as limiting services to national or regional (as opposed to local) centers, managing waiting times, developing evidence-based practice guidelines, and designing integrated approaches to care. The results of these consensus conferences were then distributed to the public in a document that called for responses from groups and individuals. Public input, then, informed service evaluation work and guideline development in the next few years.

In 1997, *The Best of Health 3* (NHC, 1997) was published. It moved public debate from the general question about whether rationing was needed, and what principles should be used, to a focus on processes for setting priorities among publicly funded services. Three points emphasized in this document made the convergence with efforts in the Nordic countries more apparent: processes for rationing decisions must be transparent; communities must be involved; and transparent tools, including guidelines and priority criteria, should be used. The public discussion of these elements of fair process is continuing as some new elements are added.

In 1998, a national Health Funding Authority (HFA) was formed and charged with responsibility for purchasing the full range of personal health, public health, and disability services for citizens. The HFA set up a wholly owned company, the Pharmaceutical Management Agency (PHARMAC) to manage its formulary. A prioritization process involving consultation with various stakeholders was established, but so far it has focused on consultation with organizations and professionals and not with community groups (Bloomfield, 2001). As a result of the consultation process, some very general principles governing priorities were adopted, among them, a special concern for reducing the health disparities between Maori and other segments of the population. PHARMAC has been successful in reducing public expenditure on pharmaceuticals at a time when most countries face rising costs.

Despite the clarity of the prioritization process, technology assessment remains advisory and does not determine decisions about coverage and dissemination. As in other countries, too few assessments can be done in a timely enough fashion to affect dissemination decisions, and it is difficult to judge which technologies on the horizon are the most important to evaluate. PHARMAC, however, generally has better access to more timely information and more control over coverage than similar agencies elsewhere. Its decisions can be appealed (but not with much success) and lobbying in Parliament has led to some changes in coverage (Bloomfield, 2001).

The New Zealand story is more advanced in some respects than others: there has been much public discussion, and the technology assessment and prioritization process in the publicly funded portion of the system tends to rest on public criteria, though these have not been examined for relevance by all stakeholders, especially community groups. Informal processes, rather than formal appeals processes, are the general rule, leaving much room for improvement. The private sector in New Zealand falls short with regard to our Publicity, Relevance, and Revisability or Appeals Conditions. The introduction of accountability for reasonableness is significant in the public sector, but still has areas where improvement is necessary.

SOME BRITISH LESSONS

The British, as we noted earlier, did not appeal to the forum of a national commission to begin a discussion of how to ration beneficial medical services. Perhaps, that is, in part, because the National Health Service (NHS) has no legal way of denying medically beneficial services, at least according to its charter. The lack of a public commission approach may also result from a well-entrenched culture encouraging implicit forms of limit setting rather than more explicit ones. Beginning a public discussion would draw heat to the politicians responsible for revising the NHS charter rather than allowing the forms of implicit rationing to deflect controversy from more central authorities.

The lack of a government-led discussion through a national commission, however, has not prevented others from raising issues concerning priority setting addressed by the Nordic commissions. The Rationing Agenda Group of the King's Fund Policy Institute, for example, challenged the public "denial of British governments of all parties . . . that health care is rationed in the NHS. . . . It has always been [rationed]: doctors and nurses have been faced with hard choices about whom to treat, in what order, and how to treat them" (New, 1997, p.2). Reorganization of the NHS by the Thatcher government, however, had the effect of making "rationing decisions more visible, since the dialogue between those commissioning care (whether they are health authorities or GPs) and those providing it is partly about interrelationships between levels of service and costs." As a result of these organizational changes, more attention has been paid at the level of district health authorities and general practitioner fundholders to the principles and process that should govern various forms of rationing.

Highly visible cases of treatment denials have also brought the issue of rationing into the public consciousness. Perhaps the most famous of these, the case of Jaymee Bowen, or Child B, can illustrate the forces that have helped focus British thinking on key elements of accountability for reasonableness (Ham and Pickard, 1998). Jaymee Bowen was given a bone marrow transplant in 1994 for acute myeloid leukemia, but the cancer returned in early 1995. Her father then requested a further experimental treatment, funding for which was denied by the

Cambridge and Huntingdon Health Authority. The experimental treatment was then funded through private donations while legal challenges to the Health Authority ruling were pursued. The first legal ruling ordered the Health Authority to fund the treatment on the grounds that it failed to pay enough attention to exceptions, that is, to distinctive features of the specific patient, and because it did not adequately weigh the importance of the European convention on human rights when it vaguely invoked resource limits. An appeals court overruled the initial decision, saying that adequate attention had been paid to exceptions and to the realities of resource limitations.

Although the Health Authority's decision was upheld in the courts, it was clear that better attention could have been paid to an explicit discussion of the grounds for its decision. To the public, it was never clear whether this was a medical decision, based on features of the specific case and judgments about appropriate treatment, or whether resource limits were an influence on the decision as well. The most detailed analysis of the case drew the conclusion that Health Authorities must "discuss and agree to values to guide decision-making . . . debating what these values mean and testing them in both hypothetical and real cases . . . clarify the process for making decisions on priorities . . . ensure that the decision-making process is robust and enables relevant options to be examined . . . provide patients with direct access to a designated decision-maker within the health authority . . . give reasons for decisions to fund or not fund treatment, explaining the basis of these decisions in order to demonstrate the legitimacy of the process, [and its] . . . consistency and fairness . . . establish an appeal mechanism to enable patients and their families to question and challenge decisions . . . ensure that effective arrangements are in place . . . for explaining the authority's position to the media and public" (Ham and Pickard, 1998, pp. 89–90).

The essentials of accountability for reasonableness show up not only in the preceding analysis by health policy experts but in a growing body of practices involving health authority and other local decision-making. For example, after its refusal of growth hormone treatment to a young child attracted national attention, Bromley Health Authority set up a working group to develop a values framework on which decision-making about individual and contractual care could take place. Responses to a survey emphasized the importance of promoting clarity about the process of decision-making, the need for adequate and timely evidence, and the guarantee of transparency for decisions about priorities (Report to Health Authority, 1997). Patient organizations and all levels of staff were then involved in drawing up the values statement. The goal was to ensure consistency and to promote accountability to those affected by decisions. Transparency and consistency were to be assured by adopting a standard format for decisions in which the written discussions would explicitly address all elements of the values framework, and these written discussions would then be the framework for subsequent debate. Deci-

sions were to be informed by legal and technical guidance, input from all stakeholders, evidence about benefit, and a careful survey of the implications and consequences of the decision.

Oxfordshire Health Authority has made its priority setting more explicit over
recent years. Though initially the Oxfordshire authority intended to be purely evidence driven in its analysis of the relative merits of various treatments, it "recognized the complexity of the process, the poverty of comparable data, and hence the
need to focus on the process of priority setting itself" (Griffiths, Reynolds &
Hope, 2000). The process developed involves a subcommittee of the Health Authority called the Priorities Forum, with a membership representative of various
interests, including the public. It addresses decisions about new drugs, new treatments, and exceptional individual needs, and its deliberations are widely distributed to interested parties.

The Priorities Forum developed an ethical framework and used it as a basis for
a "case law" approach to its decisions. The dissemination of the case law results
meant that the Forum would not have to be involved in all decisions. Other parties
could use the growing body of cases to make consistent decisions that rested on
similar evidence and reasons.

The Priorities Forum very explicitly addresses issues of resource constraints,
asking clinicians, for example, to try to specify how trade-offs against other uses
of resources should be made, or how thresholds could be set up for the use of certain treatments. The values framework also explicitly involves consideration of
resource limits. It includes considerations of effectiveness, equity, and patient
choice. The consideration of effectiveness involves four elements: effectiveness
(does the treatment achieve a desired effect?), value to the patient relative to the
value of other treatments, impact (value weighted for degree of effectiveness), and
efficiency (impact per unit cost).

The equity consideration is stated as a formal principle, requiring that similar
cases be treated similarly. It includes, however, a presumption against discrimination on the grounds of age, employment status, family circumstances, life style,
and learning disability. The equity principle also must be reconciled with two
competing considerations: maximizing population health within an available
budget and giving priority to those most in need. Neither consideration can be pursued to the exclusion of the other. In effect, this is a recognition of the inadequacy
of principled solutions to addressing the priorities and aggregation problems noted
in earlier chapters. The Forum addresses this problem by considering the cost-
effectiveness of the intervention (using a quality-adjusted life year approach to
measure effectiveness). If the intervention is less effective than those normally
funded, it then asks if there are special considerations that might involve important issues of distributive fairness. For example, population health might be made
secondary to evaluating the urgency of the need, whether the treatment was for

someone with seriously compromised quality of life, or whether the extra cost was the result of patient characteristics that should not affect priority.

The value of patient choice addresses several distinct issues. Outcome measures should include factors that matter to patients; patients should have choices among funded services. There must be room to look at the individual features of a specific patient and not judge exceptional cases by crude averages.

The Oxfordshire Forum uses this value framework and, for many types of rationing decisions, publishes explicit reports on its deliberations. One common type is the evaluation of new drugs for the formulary. Though these kinds of decisions were initially forced upon the Authority by the market reforms in the NHS in the early '90s, they now clearly go beyond cost containment and involve value decisions regarding choices between prevention, treatment, and other kinds of care. The Forum is considering how to involve the public in open discussion about these matters.

Just as Oxfordshire has had to move beyond considerations of efficacy and efficiency in its deliberations about new drugs and treatments, so too have some Canadian efforts. Committees deliberating about the allocation of cardiac care resources, pharmacy benefits, and home health services have all begun to attend to the transparency of their deliberations and have made, in varying degrees, an effort to involve more stakeholders in their decisions. (Singer, Martin, Giacomini & Purdy, 2000).

Although some NHS health authorities have introduced key elements of accountability for reasonableness in their decision-making process, on the whole, the approach countrywide has been ad hoc (Robert & Ham, 2001). A bright spot in the national story is the introduction of the National Institute for Clinical Excellence (NICE). It is intended to give more systematic recommendations about clinical benefits and costs to the secretary of state. Specifically, it carries out technology assessment, develops and disseminates clinical guidelines, and oversees clinical audits and confidential inquiries. Like technology assessment organizations in other contexts, its role is advisory, and without knowing just how actual coverage decisions are then made, it is difficult to confer the legitimacy achieved in the technology assessment process itself to the actual coverage and dissemination decisions that are made. Even NICE, however, has not engaged members of the public in a process of evaluating criteria for their relevance; this has primarily been the task of experts. Though NICE embodies key elements of accountability for reasonableness, these conditions on fair process have a long way to go before they filter into the many levels of decision-making in the British system.

In contrast to the Nordic countries, the Netherlands, or New Zealand, neither Britain nor Canada has had a government-led discussion of priority setting or rationing. Indeed, in Britain, there is some public pretense that true rationing does not happen. Still, nongovernmental debate has focused attention on rationing, and the British reforms early in the decade have focused attention on local health authority decisions, especially when there are visible denials of treatment, as in the Child B and Bromley cases. To achieve acceptability and legitimacy for these forms of local limit setting, local authorities have adopted key elements of accountability for reasonableness, as have national programs in the Nordic countries and New Zealand. With different starting points, then, there has been convergence on similar solutions.

ACCOUNTABILITY AND LIMIT-SETTING IN DEVELOPING COUNTRIES

In developing countries, where both public and private resources available for health care are more limited, accountability for reasonableness in decisions remains crucial to establishing the legitimacy of priority setting and health reforms. In the brief remarks that follow, we draw on work in progress in four developing countries (Mexico, Colombia, Thailand, Pakistan) carried out by one of us (Daniels, Bryant, Castano, et al., 2000). The project aims at adapting a policy tool, the "benchmarks of fairness for health care reform," from its original application for proposed U.S. reforms in 1993 into something useful in developing countries.

A remarkable result of this project is that there is convergence on nine benchmarks of fairness, with many specific operational criteria for each benchmark, despite the huge cultural and historical and political differences among these countries (Daniels, Bryant, Castano, et al., 2000). In all four sites, there was agreement on the importance of evaluating the forms of accountability introduced through health system reform. Without accountability, including accountability for reasonableness with respect to priority-setting and limit-setting decisions, little reform takes place and great cynicism results.

Much of the discussion of accountability for reasonableness in this book, which focuses in part on coverage decisions for new, expensive technologies and treatments, sounds esoteric, even precious, in light of the kinds of resource allocation decisions that must be made in many developing countries. Nevertheless, because the decisions forced by the much greater scarcity in developing countries are so profound in their effects, accountability for reasonableness is all the more important. This conclusion can be brought out by some brief remarks about the context in which resource allocation decisions must be made in these systems.

First, it important to know that, in most developing countries, a basic structural problem in the economy shapes the problem of scarcity and thus the scope of all resource allocation decisions. In developed countries, we are accustomed to thinking about tax- and insurance-based schemes (both public and private) that assure universal coverage for a fairly comprehensive set of medical services. Limit setting takes place at the margin within such schemes. The very large informal sector of the economy in most developing countries—often 60% (as in Mexico) to 90% (as in Pakistan) of the work force—cannot be taxed or included within premium-based insurance schemes. Instead, the much smaller formal sector of the economy, which can be taxed, provides tax revenues aimed at providing medical services to the informal sector. This means that public-sector systems are poorly funded, especially when the very wealthy land and corporation owners, as in Pakistan, control enough of the political process to keep themselves from being taxed. It is possible to construct a social-security- or employer-based insurance system for the formal sector, but this usually involves significant tiering of benefits between the sectors.

In theory, public-sector services are supposed to meet various levels of need, from primary to tertiary care, for all those without formal insurance. In reality, these systems usually fall far short of doing so, both because they are underfunded and because they are often riddled with bureaucratic inefficiency and corruption. Doctors, for example, often collect public sector salaries but are really only "shadow providers" who actually see patients in private clinics for cash.

One common reform strategy—implemented in Mexico and Colombia, but put on hold in Thailand—is to reform the public sector so that it actually delivers universal access to at least a defined, minimum benefit package. Successive reforms may broaden that benefit package. Other aspects of reform would then regulate the quality and effectiveness of services provided for cash in the private sector.

Accountability for reasonableness has a central role in the deliberations about the benefit package that should be included in such reform efforts, both in an initial reform and in successive stages. It requires that rationales for the scope of the package and its successive improvements be explicit, and that relevant considerations be made explicit, including the real limits on access that result from private resources being used for other services.

A second focus of recent health system reforms has been the attempt to integrate and strengthen formal-sector insurance systems, both social security and private. Here, too, great variation within one country usually exists in the levels of benefits among different insurance schemes. Some systems include dependents of workers and others do not; some have more, or less, inclusive drug benefits. Accountability for reasonableness has a key role in opening the deliberation about the effects of reforms of this part of the system to broader public discussion.

A third central focus of recent health system reforms has been aimed at curing the bureaucratic inefficiency that haunts large ministries of health. External non-governmental organizations, including the World Bank, have pushed hard to introduce decentralization and local autonomy into the administrative structures. In many cases, this is coupled with efforts to promote increased use of a private sector. Decentralization and increased autonomy usually take the form of allowing district health boards or hospital boards to act as fundholders, who are then responsible for working within budgets they control.

Accountability for reasonableness is key to making these strategies effective. Without building into the reform the requirements of transparency, open deliberation about relevant considerations, and appeals of decisions, there is no way to ensure that decentralization or increased local autonomy will actually improve resource allocation decisions at all. Those pilot efforts—in Thailand and Pakistan, for example—that have proved most promising are ones in which there was increased transparency in the workings of public and private institutions and increased involvement of community groups in them.

A central point behind accountability for reasonableness is the educative role it plays, and the opportunity it provides to improve deliberation at various levels within these institutions. In developing countries, there is often very little developed civil society in the form of advocacy groups representing interests that transcend local communities and unite subgroups among them. Improving and empowering such elements of civic society is key to improving accountability in general. The specific elements of accountability for reasonableness provide information that enhances this process of developing civil society.

A particular institutional form contributing to that kind of development is an accessible, functioning appeals process. A universal issue in the four countries involved in the benchmarks project is the absence of developed appeals mechanisms for resolving disputes about treatment or coverage decisions or other failures of the health care system. The absence of such mechanisms breeds cynicism and a reduced willingness to engage the system in efforts at change.

In the benchmarks project, considerable attention was focused on community participation as a central feature of the criteria for fairness. There is considerable evidence that, without community involvement, many plans for reform are simply bureaucratic fantasies that cannot be implemented. Similarly, the evaluation of health system reforms must include input from communities the reforms are aimed at. In many contexts, direct community involvement is the only causally effective check on otherwise unresponsive bureaucracies and the only way to make sure that particular arguments and considerations are directly addressed.

Though accountability for reasonableness is aimed at improving democratic deliberation, and though that sometimes means that direct involvement of communities in planning and evaluation is necessary, there is no general requirement that direct, participatory democracy has to play a role at every level within the institutions that make decisions. In considering how to make health plans in the United States responsive to patient needs, some people advocate direct consumer participation in decision-making. Though this may in some cases improve deliberation and reduce distrust, it is not generally feasible and can simply lead to tokenism and co-optation. Though direct community participation often improves responsiveness and the quality of deliberation, it is neither a necessary nor sufficient condition for assuring accountability for reasonableness (Daniels & Sabin, 1998b).

Sen (1999) has remarked that democratic process is of crucial importance in development not only because of its *intrinsic* value as a form of freedom, and not only because of its *instrumental* role as a way of addressing broader needs and interests, but also because of its *constructive* function in developing understanding and the conceptual apparatus to address challenging public issues. Accountability for reasonableness, by enhancing public deliberation, empowers people in ways that improve this constructive function of democracy.

CROSS NATIONAL LEARNING ABOUT FAIR PROCESS

Several points emerge from our brief look at international examples. First, how explicitly countries are willing to address the problem of scarcity and the limits to care varies considerably. The United States, with the exception of Oregon, has been quite unwilling to raise the issue through government-led initiatives. Specific features of American political culture, such as the growing prominence in American public debate of libertarian ideas about individual choice, reflected in the concept of insurance based on individual medical savings accounts, stand in the way of clarity about collective problems. The Nordic countries and New Zealand have adopted the opposite approach. The British fall in the middle. There is value to the public discussion where it has taken place, but a refusal to have the publicly led discussion at the systemwide level does not, as the British and American examples show, preclude progress at other levels.

Second, despite variations in the starting point of discussions, there is evidence of convergence on some necessary elements of a solution to the problem of how to ration fairly and establish legitimacy for the results. The key ideas that we have called accountability for reasonableness—transparency about the grounds for decisions, the appeal to reasons that people agree are relevant, a process of appeals—have emerged as parts of the U.S. debate about managed care regulation, the Norwegian and New Zealand discussions of fair process, and practical steps taken by British health authorities.

Third, the fact of this convergence on fair process at the level of decentralized decision-making, whether in the private U.S. system or in the public authorities in Britain and elsewhere, suggests that the kind of reasonable moral disagreement about cases that is endemic to rationing requires a mechanism encouraging deliberation and its input into a broader democratic process.

Fourth, if these points are correct, then there is an emerging agenda for research and policy development. It is necessary to examine efforts to implement fair rationing procedures across national boundaries. The many factors that would discourage such efforts, such as the conviction that political and health system differences between countries vitiate efforts at transferring experiences, must be set aside. Too much is at stake not to engage in a serious effort at examining best practices across variations in system design.

Finally, the examples of convergence on key elements of accountability for reasonableness give content to the idea, discussed earlier, that there is a middle path between calls for explicit and implicit rationing. Some efforts at implementing fair process call for articulating a set of values or an ethics framework of the sort we noted in Bromley Health or Oxfordshire, but this framework is not the same thing as the articulation of explicit criteria for rationing, as by specifying a method of cost-effectiveness analysis and a range of acceptable values. Explicit criteria would give specific outcomes for rationing without further ethical deliberation, whereas an ethical-framework approach requires that such deliberation take place. By treating these decisions as precedents that create a form of case law, something akin to the criteria invoked in explicit rationing efforts will emerge over time. In this way the "middle path" draws on the strengths of both implicit and explicit approaches to rationing. Over time, careful deliberation about the specifics of particular decisions becomes coupled with articulation of transparent grounds for further decisions.

11

LEARNING TO SHARE
MEDICAL RESOURCES

Under what conditions should the public accept limits to care as fair and legitimate?

This is the central question guiding our inquiry in this book. To motivate discussion of the question, we have argued that justice requires setting reasonable and fair limits to care but that general principles of distributive justice fail to provide us with a clear way to resolve important disputes about the fairness of limits. Because of the resulting unavoidable moral controversy, distrust often surrounds both public and private institutions that make practical, limit-setting decisions. Trust and legitimacy are international problems and not simply a function of the U.S. system of competitive managed care. In the absence of consensus on appropriate distributive principles, a process for decision-making that all can accept as fair is crucial to dispelling distrust. Then, the outcomes of the fair process should be acceptable as fair and legitimate.

We have characterized key elements of the fair process by describing four conditions that must be met: the Publicity, Relevance, Revision and Appeals, and Enforcement Conditions that constitute accountability for reasonableness. Conformance with some of these principles is a feature of best practices in a variety of public and private institutions. Nevertheless, efforts to reform these institutions, such as the reform proposals regarding regulation of managed care in the United States, lack a coherent grasp and commitment to accountability for reasonableness, even as they embody some elements of it.

Still, as the illustrations we have provided show, accountability for reasonableness is an achievable goal, provided we have a coherent grasp of what it involves and the political will to implement it. It is not pie in the sky nor is it utopian. It does require reform with teeth.

Proving it is not utopian, however, requires addressing a question that is part of our claim that accountability for reasonableness is central to fairness and legitimacy. That question asks for the conditions under which the public *should* accept limits as fair and legitimate. What exactly is involved in this normative claim? Clarifying this point will help us answer, as well, the question in our subtitle for the book, "Can we learn to share medical resources?"

It is a commonplace—sometimes a misleading one—of ethical theory and ethical reasoning that *ought* implies *can*. For us to be obliged to do something, it must be possible for us to do it. If the public should, or ought to, accept the results of a fair process as fair and legitimate limits, it must be possible—psychologically, socially, culturally—for it to view those results in the appropriate way. In other words, the public must understand the need for such limits, the reasons for relying on fair process, the kinds of reasons that are appropriate for setting such limits, and the procedures for challenging decisions and engaging in deliberation and debate about them. In short, the public should accept such conditions when it can accept them, and it can accept them only when it understands them and the need for them.

Only a public that has gone through a sustained educational process will be equipped to accept the fairness and legitimacy of limits. Yet, accountability for reasonableness itself helps to establish the conditions under which such an education can take place. It provides the material that can move the public along a social learning curve, improving its grasp of the need for limits and the appropriate grounds and conditions for making decisions about them. For example, the value of the Publicity and Relevance conditions, we have suggested, is the "case law" they establish regarding limit setting over time. That case law familiarizes people with appropriate reasons and sets standards for reasoning about similar cases. A transparent and responsive process of revision and appeal similarly contributes to a grasp of the kinds of reasons that appropriately shape policy decisions and exceptions to them.

Have we set up a paradox? Which comes first, the chicken or the egg? The public cannot, and therefore is not obliged to, accept the results of the process as fair and legitimate unless it understands the need for limits and the types of reasons that should play a role in setting them. Lacking that grasp, there seems to be no reason why the public should institute accountability for reasonableness. Yet accountability for reasonableness helps provide the experience through which public understanding of limits can grow and thus sets the stage for better democratic deliberation about the design and management of a health care system.

Fortunately, the paradox is overstated. Imperfect processes can improve our grasp of what better processes would be. As with many aspects of real life, we pull ourselves up by our own bootstraps, using imperfect understanding and learning from experience to generate better understanding. We do not want to leave the point with this sort of general answer, however, and instead want to conclude by saying a bit more about how the process of social learning can take place as we move institutions in the direction of accountability for reasonableness.

In the preceding chapter, we discussed the fact that public debate in some European countries was stimulated by the establishment of national commissions on priority setting. In contrast, in the United States, with the exception of Oregon, there has been a denial by both public and private institutions that anything like rationing ever goes on in our system.

One intriguing American exception is the recent Supreme Court decision in Pegram v. Herdrich (120 S. Ct. 2143), in which Justice David Souter remarked that "inducement to ration care is the very point of any HMO scheme, and rationing necessarily raises some risks while reducing others." Justice Souter then commented that drawing "a line between good and bad HMOs would embody a judgment about socially acceptable medical risk that would turn on facts not readily accessible to courts and on social judgments not wisely required of courts unless resort cannot be had to the legislature." Since the plaintiff in this case had argued that rationing was taking place, it was perhaps necessary that Justice Souter acknowledged it as well. A more generous interpretation is that some public learning had been taking place as a result of the debate about managed care. Still, the Court unanimously threw the problem of finding an acceptable way to carry out rationing back to the legislature—ducking, perhaps correctly, the onus of grappling with the line-drawing problems that must be faced somewhere in the system.

Obviously, societies that share health care resources in a collectively designed system must face public debate about limits in a way that Americans can, at least temporarily, dodge. This fact creates an obstacle to public education in the United States. Public debate and the attempt to arrive at national consensus through commissions is an important contribution to societal learning.

Nevertheless, public learning can take place even in the absence of the kind of public debate that surrounds national commissions. Ironically, the very fact that the American system has built greater distrust of private limit setters than exists in many publicly administered systems has led to more discussion and education about limit setting at the institutional level. The exemplary practices we described in earlier chapters show some American leadership in managing the debate at this level.

Other recent practices of some health plans explicitly aim at both transparency and education. Harvard Pilgrim Health Care in Massachusetts is putting the minutes of its organizational ethics program meetings on the Web. Allina Health System in Minnesota has published an extended statement of principles that focuses on the necessity of trade-offs among values. The Group Health Cooperative in Washington State has held public forums on complicated, real-world rationing issues. Blue Cross Blue Shield of Tennessee has published rationales for its policies on its Web site. United Health has announced a "no surprises" approach in which it plans to extend the openness and transparency of its policies. Merck-Medco Managed Care, one of the largest pharmacy benefit management companies, is also publishing evidence and rationales for its benefits design features, including formulary restrictions, on its Web site. The learning curve stimulated by these measures affects both clinicians and patients.

Full implementation of accountability for reasonableness would do far more. As we argued in Chapter 4, the involvement of all stakeholders—especially consumers—makes publicity a reality, enriches deliberation about what counts as relevant reasons, and creates potential for a robust process of revisions and appeals. In itself, stakeholder participation does not necessarily make decisions more democratic or provide a vehicle for consent to limits. By itself, it does not create legitimacy. Rather, by enhancing accountability for reasonableness, and especially by pursuing it as its goal, stakeholder participation enhances legitimacy. Enhanced by such participation, accountability for reasonableness contributes in multiple, often indirect, ways to the deliberative quality of broader democratic processes that are ultimately responsible for regulating the fairness of the health system.

It is worth tracing the routes through which accountability for reasonableness contributes to broader democratic deliberation. Imagine a system that fully implemented such accountability in the various institutions responsible for allocating and delivering health care. Learning about limits and how to establish them fairly would then take place where health plans and other provider organizations interact with various stakeholders—clinicians, employers, managers, and patients. Through proper institutional support, learning would take place within the doctor–patient relationship—a point we return to shortly. Societal learning would take place as a result of these institutional interactions with specific stakeholders and more broadly in the aggregate. This learning would infuse in various ways into the process of deliberation that takes place in an array of democratic institutions: legislative and executive bodies, the courts, and private associations, including professional associations and private regulative bodies such as the National Committee for Quality Assurance. We assume the quality of deliberation in these bodies would improve, as would the outcomes of deliberation—legal supervision, government regulation, and self-regulation. Accountability for reasonableness is the mechanism through which this learning would be facilitated and improved deliberation made more feasible.

It is worth singling out for special attention the learning that takes place within the doctor–patient relationship, for it may have the greatest impact on the public's grasp of the need for fair limits and the grounds for establishing them. Accountability for reasonableness prepares the way for full development of collaborative decision-making about treatments between patients and doctors. This model of the doctor–patient relationship has emerged over the last few decades as the dominant model of proper decision-making about treatments. The collaborative model opens the way to the mutual education of doctor and patient, and accountability for reasonableness provides some of the institutional supports needed for it.

In the early 1990s, clinicians in mental health at the then Harvard Community Health Plan, with the advice of the population they served, decided to offer more outpatient care to their sickest patients (Sabin, 1998b). Although the budget for care was not increased, these clinicians allowed to reorder their service's priorities. They concluded they could increase services to the sickest patients only by requiring a new payment from the less sick after their eighth outpatient appointment. (As a practical matter, they thus accepted the budget limits on mental health care as fixed; perhaps, in a system that more fairly allocated resources across broader parts of the health care budget, the particular reallocation described here might not have been necessary.)

After they made this change, clinicians discussed the new policy with their patients. With patients who were eligible for more services, they said something like this: "The bad news, as we know, is that you have the misfortune of suffering from a severe illness (e.g., schizophrenia). The good news is that we now have more outpatient treatment resources available to us." With their healthier patients, who had previously not had to make a payment after eight outpatient sessions, they had the opposite conversation: "The good news is that, even though you have some significant problems, you do not have a severe illness like schizophrenia or manic depression. The bad news is that, after eight sessions, there is now a new fee." No one was happy about paying the new fee. But almost no one thought the policy was unfair.

The clinicians did not explain the priority system by presenting cost-effectiveness analyses or complex ethical arguments. They used simple commonsense terms that made fundamental human sense. The policy had the same kind of obvious reasonableness as when a clinician has to interrupt an appointment with one patient to attend to an emergency with another.

To support priorities and rationing, clinicians must be able to see the policy rationale with the same emotional clarity and immediacy with which they see their individual patient's needs. To explain the policy, they must be able to put it in simple terms that do not presuppose university degrees in economics or philosophy. To do either, institutions must be more open about the rationales for their policies and rely on rationales that all can see are relevant. These elements of accountability for reasonableness thus provide institutional support for the mutual learning encouraged by collaborative decision-making.

The example of the changed fee structure for mental health care at one health plan illustrates a related point, one essential to making collaborative decision-making deliver the education about limits we have been discussing. The example illustrates a crucial change in the advocacy role of the clinician. These clinicians had to see themselves as advocates for their own patients but also as advocates working with the goal of delivering health care fairly to a population. They had to balance these tasks and communicate their perception of priorities to all their patients, those who benefited and those who lost as a result of the policy change.

These clinicians were still advocates for their patients, but they became "proportional advocates" not "traditional patient advocates" (Pearson, 2000). The traditional advocate thinks only of the dyadic relation between one patient and one doctor, with the result that such dyads compete for resources in ways that may well lead to outcomes that are worse for population health and unfair to some patients. Proportional advocacy involves a new understanding of professional obligations—it requires physicians to act as advocates for the fair delivery of health to a population, balancing various interests that may compete. We made this same point in Chapter 8 when we argued that physician incentives should balance the multiple interests involved in meeting needs fairly.

This new understanding on the part of clinicians emerged in the Harvard Community Health Plan case through consultation with a range of doctors and patients within one health plan. Accountability for reasonableness encourages the conditions under which such consultation, mutual learning, and mutual support are provided by health plans or public agencies that deliver care under resource constraints. With this kind of institutional support, in publicly or privately administered systems, the social learning curve improves.

The various levels at which social learning takes place clearly interact and reinforce each other. As we noted, where national political leadership takes a role in initiating public discussion, understanding within the clinical relationship can be improved. But, as we have tried to emphasize, political leadership, while desirable, is not essential to progress. As the public understands more through these institutional policies and interaction with doctors in the system, public debate can itself be enriched. The result will then be a better democratic deliberation about how fair process can be implemented at all necessary levels. Regulation will be aimed at supporting such fair process, not at mandating the specifics of health care delivery. Accountability for reasonableness facilitates this democratic process by supporting the conditions under which it is possible and likely to be most effective.

References

Albert, R.K., Lewis, S., Wood, D., et al. (1996). Economic aspects of lung volume reduction surgery. *Chest* 110:1068–71.

American Medical Association. (1998). Council for Ethical and Judicial Affairs. *Opinion* 8.03 (Conflicts of Interest).

Anderson, E. (1999). What is the point of equality? *Ethics* 109:287–337.

Arneson, R.J. (1988). Equality and equal opportunity for welfare. *Philosophical Studies* 54:79–95.

Arrow, K. (1963). Uncertainty and the welfare economics of medical care. *American Economic Review* 53:941–73.

Bayer, R. (1989). *Private Acts, Social Consequences: AIDS and the Politics of Public Health.* New York: Free Press.

Beebe, D.B., Rosenfeld, A.B., & Collins, N. (1997). An approach to decisions about coverage of investigational treatments. *HMO Practice* 11(2): 65–67.

Berwick, D.M. (1996). Payment by capitation and the quality of care. *New England Journal of Medicine* 335(16):1227–31.

Bezwoda, W.R., Seymour, L., & Dansey, R.D. (1995). High-dose chemotherapy with hematopoietic rescue as primary treatment for metastatic breast cancer: A randomized trial. *Journal of Clinical Oncology* 13:2483–89.

Blendon, R.J., Brodie, M., Benson, J.M., et al. (1998). Understanding the managed care backlash. *Health Affairs* 17(4):80–94.

Bloomfield, A. (2001). New Zealand. In Ham, C. & Robert, G. *The next phase of priority setting in health care: Securing fairness and legitimacy.* Unpublished manuscript.

Bodenheimer, T.S. & Grumbach, K. (1996). Capitation or decapitation: Keeping your head in changing times. *Journal of the American Medical Association* 276(8):1025–32.

Boorse, C. (1975). On the distinction between disease and illness. *Philosophy & Public Affairs* 5(1):49–68.

Boorse, C. (1976). What a theory of mental health should be. *Journal of the Theory of Social Behavior* 6(1):61–84.

Boorse, C. (1977). Health as a theoretical concept. *Philosophy of Science* 44:542–73.

Boorse, C. (1997). A rebuttal on health. In Humber, J.M. & Almeder, R.F. (Eds.) *What is Disease?* Totowa, NJ: Humana Press, pp. 1–134.

Boorse, C. (in press). A rebuttal on functions. In Ariew, A., Cummins, R. & Perlman, M. (Eds.) *Functions: New Readings in the Philosophy of Psychology and Biology.* New York: Oxford University Press.

Brantigan, O.C., Mueller, E., & Kress, M.B. (1959). A surgical approach to pulmonary emphysema. *American Review of Respiratory Disease* 80:194–206 (Suppl).

Brock, D. (1988). Ethical issues in recipient selection for organ transplantation. In Mathieu, D. (Ed.) *Organ Substitution Technology: Ethical, Legal, and Public Policy Issues.* Boulder, CO: Westview Press, pp. 86–99.

Brock, D. (1998). Ethical issues in the development of summary measures of health status. In Institute of Medicine, *Summarizing population health: Directions for the development and application of population metrics.* Washington DC: National Academy Press, pp. 73–86.

Brock, D. & Daniels, N. (1994). Ethical foundations of the Clinton administration's proposed health care system. *Journal of the American Medical Association* 271: 1189–96.

Buchanan, A., Brock, D., Daniels, N., & Wikler, D. (2000). *From Chance to Choice: Genetics and Justice.* New York: Cambridge University Press.

Bullen, B. (1998) *What is a prudent purchaser?* Available from: National Association of State Medicaid Directors, 810 First Street NE (Suite 500), Washington DC 20002–4267.

Calabresi, G. & Bobbitt, P. (1978). *Tragic Choices.* New York: Norton.

Cangialose, C.B., Cary, S.J., Hoffman, L.H., & Ballard, D.J. (1997). Impact of managed care on quality of healthcare: Theory and evidence. *American Journal of Managed Care* 3:1153–70.

Cohen, G.A. (1989) On the currency of egalitarian justice. *Ethics* 99:906–44.

Cohen, J. (1994). Pluralism and proceduralism. *Chicago-Kent Law Review* 69(3):589–618.

Cohen, J. (1996a). Procedure and Substance in Deliberative Democracy. In Benhabib, S. (Ed.). *Democracy and Difference: Changing Boundaries of the Political.* Princeton, NJ: Princeton University Press. pp. 95–119.

Cohen, J. (1996b) Deliberative democracy. Unpublished manuscript.

Cooper, J.D. & Lefrak, S.S. (1996). "Is volume reduction surgery appropriate in the treatment of emphysema? . . . Yes." *American Journal of Respiratory and Critical Care Medicine* 153(4):1201–04.

Cooper, J.D. & Patterson, G.A. (1996). Lung volume reduction surgery for severe emphysema. *Seminars in Thoracic and Cardiovascular Surgery* 8(1): 52–60.

Cooper, J.D., Trulock, E.P., Triantafillou, A.N., et al. (1996). Bilateral pneumectomy (volume reduction) for chronic obstructive pulmonary disease. *Journal of Thoracic and Cardiovascular Surgery* 109(1):106–19.

Coulter, A. & Ham, C. (Eds.) 2000. *The Global Challenge of Health Care Rationing.* Philadelphia: Open University Press.

Cykert, S., Hanson, C., Layson, R., & Joines, J. (1997). Primary care physicians and capitated reimbursement. *Journal General Internal Medicine* 12:192–94.

Daniels, N. (1985). *Just Health Care.* New York: Oxford University Press.

Daniels, N. (1986). Why saying "no" to patients in the United States is so hard: cost containment, justice and provider autonomy. *New England Journal of Medicine* 314: 1381–83.

Daniels, N. (1988). Justice and the dissemination of big ticket technologies. In Mathieu, D. *Organ Substitution Technology: Ethical, Legal, and Public Policy Issues.* Boulder, CO: Westview. pp. 211–20.

Daniels, N. (1991). Is the Oregon rationing plan fair? *Journal of the American Medical Association* 265:2232–35.

Daniels, N. (1992). Growth hormone therapy for short stature: Can we support the treatment/enhancement distinction? *Growth: Genetics and Hormones* 8(2):46–48 (Suppl).

Daniels, N. (1993). Rationing fairly: programmatic considerations. *Bioethics* 7(2/3): 224–33.

Daniels, N. (1995). *Seeking Fair Treatment: From the AIDS Epidemic to National Health Care Reform.* New York: Oxford University Press.

Daniels, N. (1996). *Justice and Justification: Reflective Equilibrium in Theory and Practice.* New York: Cambridge University Press.

Daniels, N. (1998a). Rationing medical care: a philosopher's perspective on outcomes and process. *Economics and Philosophy* 14:27–50.

Daniels, N. (1998b). Kamm's moral methods. *Philosophy and Phenomenological Research* 58:947–54.

Daniels, N. (1999). Enabling Democratic Deliberation: How Managed Care Organizations Ought to Make Decisions about Coverage for New Technologies. In Macedo, S. (Ed.). *Deliberative Politics: Essays on Democracy and Disagreement.* New York: Oxford University Press, pp. 198–210.

Daniels, N. (2000). Accountability for reasonableness. *British Medical Journal* 321: 1300–01.

Daniels, N. (2002). Democratic equality: Rawls' complex egalitarianism. In Freeman, S., *Companion to Rawls.* Oxford: Blackwells (in press).

Daniels, N., Bryant, J., Castano, R.A., et al. (June, 2000) Benchmarks of fairness for health care reform: A policy tool for developing countries. *WHO Bulletin* 78(6):740–50.

Daniels, N., Kennedy, B., & Kawachi, I. (1999). Why justice is good for our health: Social determinants of health inequalities. *Daedalus* 128(4):215–51.

Daniels, N., Kennedy, B., & Kawachi, I. (2000). *Is Inequality Bad for Our Health?* Boston: Beacon Press.

Daniels, N., Light, D., & Caplan, R. (1996). *Benchmarks of Fairness for Health Care Reform.* New York: Oxford University Press.

Daniels, N. & Sabin, J.E. (1997). Limits to health care: Fair procedures, democratic deliberation, and the legitimacy problem for insurers. *Philosophy and Public Affairs* 26(4):303–50.

Daniels, N. & Sabin, J.E. (1998a). Closure, fair procedures, and setting limits within managed care organizations. *Journal of the American Geriatrics Society* 46(3):351–54.

Daniels, N. & Sabin, J.E. (1998b). The ethics of accountability and the reform of managed care organizations. *Health Affairs* 17(5):50–69.

Daniels, N. & Sabin J.E. (1998c). Last-chance therapies and managed care: pluralism, fair procedures, and legitimacy. *Hastings Center Report* 28(2):27–41.

Daniels, N. & Sabin, J.E. (2001). What is consistency and fairness in pharmacy benefits? *Medical Care* 39:312–14.

Danish Council of Ethics. (1996). *Priority-setting in the Health Service—A Report.* Copenhagen: Danish Council of Ethics.

Davies, H.T.O. (1999). Falling public trust in health services: Implications for accountability. *Journal of Health Services Research and Policy,* 4(4):193–94.

Dworkin, R. (1981). What is equality? Part I: Equality of welfare. *Philosophy & Public Affairs* 10:185–246.

Edgar, W. (2000). Rationing health care in New Zealand—How the public has a say. In Coulter, A. & Ham, C. (Eds.) *The Global Challenge of Health Care Rationing.* Philadelphia: Open University Press, pp. 175–91.

Elster, J. (1992). *Local Justice: How Institutions Allocate Scarce Goods and Necessary Burdens.* New York: Russell Sage.

Engelhardt, H.T. (1974). Disease of masturbation: Values and the concept of disease. *Bulletin of the History of Medicine* 48(2):234–48.

Estlund, D. (1997). Beyond fairness and deliberation: The epistemic dimension of democratic authority. In Bohman, J. & Rehg, W. (Eds.) *Deliberative Democracy.* Boston: MIT Press, pp. 173–204.

Finkelstein, B.S., Silvers J.B., & Marrero U. (1998). Insurance coverage, physician recommendations, and access to emerging treatments: growth hormone therapy for childhood short stature. *Journal of the American Medical Association* 279: 663–68.

Freedman, B. (1987). Equipoise and the ethics of clinical research. *New England Journal of Medicine* 317:141–45.

Friedman, M. (September 13, 1970). The social responsibility of business is to increase its profits. *New York Times Magazine,* 124–30.

Gold, M.R., Hurley, R., Lake, T., et al. (1995). A national survey of the arrangements managed care plans make with physicians. *New England Journal of Medicine* 333: 1678–83.

Gray, B.H. (1997). Trust and trustworthy care in the managed care era: Can managed care organizations take on the mantle of trust that traditionally has belonged to physicians? *Health Affairs* 16(1):34–49.

Greene, J. (February 3, 1996). County has Treatment for Lungs. *Orange County Register,* pp. 9.

Griffiths, S., Reynolds, J., & Hope, T. (2000). "Priority Setting in Practice," In Coulter, A. & Ham, C. *The Global Challenge of Health Care Rationing.* Philadelphia: Open University Press. (pp. 203–13).

Gutman, A. & Thompson, D. (1996). *Democracy and Disagreement.* Cambridge: Harvard University Press.

Hadorn, D. (1991). Setting health care priorities in Oregon: Cost-effectiveness meets the rule of rescue. *Journal of the American Medical Association* 265:2218–25.

Ham, C. & Pickard, S. (1998). *Tragic Choices in Health Care: The Case of Child B.* London: King's Fund.

Hellinger, F.J. (1996). The impact of financial incentives on physician behavior in managed care plans: A review of the evidence. *Medical Care Research and Review* 53(3): 294–314.

HHS News (April 14, 1996). Press Release.

Hillman, A.L., Pauly, M.V., & Kerstein, J.J. (1989). How do financial incentives affect physicians' clinical decisions and the financial performance of health maintenance organizations? *New England Journal of Medicine* 321:86–92.

Hillman, A.L., Pauly, M.V., Kerman, K., & Martinek, C.R. (1991). HMO managers' views on financial incentives and quality. *Health Affairs* 10(6):207–19.

Himmelstein, D.U. & Woolhandler, S. (1986). Cost without benefit: Administrative waste in U.S. health care. *New England Journal of Medicine* 315: 441–45.

Hollingsworth, E.J. & Sweeney, J.K. (1997). Mental health expenditures for services for people with severe mental illnesses. *Psychiatric Services* 48:485–90.

Holm, S. (2000). Developments in the Nordic countries—goodbye to the simple solutions. In Coulter, A. & Ham, C. (Eds.) *The Global Challenge of Health Care Rationing.* Philadelphia: Open University Press, pp. 29–37.

Institute for Clinical Systems Integration. (1995). TA # 23: *Lung Volume Reduction Surgery.*

Jecker, N.S. & Jonsen, A.R. (1997). Managed care: A house of mirrors. *Journal of Clinical Ethics* 8(3):230–41.

Josephson, G.W. & Karcz, A. (1997). The impact of physician economic incentives on admission rates of patients with ambulatory sensitive conditions: An analysis comparing two managed care structures and indemnity insurance. *American Journal of Managed Care* 3(1):49–56.

Johnsson, J. (1996). Trial focus: public unease with physician incentives. (David and Stephanie Gross vs Prudential Health Care Plan). *American Medical News* 39 (30):1–3.

Kamm, F. (1987). The choice between people, commonsense morality, and doctors. *Bioethics* 1:255–71.

Kamm, F. (1993). *Morality, Mortality: Death and Whom to Save From it:* Vol. 1. Oxford: Oxford University Press.

Kao, A., Zaslavsky, A.M., Green, D.C., et al. (2001). Physician incentives and disclosure of payment methods to patients. *Journal of General Internal Medicine,* 16:181–88.

Karasnik, A., Groenewegen, P.P., Pedersen, P.A., et al., (1990). Changing remuneration systems: Effects on activity in general practice. *British Medical Journal* 300: 1698–1701.

Kawachi, I. & Kennedy, B.P. (1999). Income inequality and health: Pathways and mechanisms. *Health Services Research* 34:215–27.

Kawachi, I., Kennedy, B.P., & Wilkinson, R. (1999) (Eds.) *Income Inequality and Health: A Reader.* New York: The New Press.

Kitzhaber, J. (1993). Rationing in action: Prioritising health services in an era of limits: The Oregon experience. *British Medical Journal* 307:373–77.

Klein, R. (1995). Priorities and rationing: Pragmatism or principles? *British Medical Journal* 311:761–62.

Klein, R., Day, P., & Redmayne, S. (1996). *Managing Scarcity: Priority Setting and Rationing in the National Health Service.* Philadelphia: Open University Press.

Knickman, J.B., Hughes, R.G., Taylor, H., et al. (1996). Tracking consumers' reactions to the changing health care system: Early indicators. *Health Affairs* 15(2):21–32.

Kuttner, R. (1998). Must good HMOs go bad? The commercialization of prepaid group health care." *New England Journal of Medicine* 338:1558–63.

Lee, A.J. (1997). The role of financial incentives in shaping clinical practice patterns and practice efficiency. *American Journal of Cardiology* 80(8B):28H–32H.

Levit, K., Cowan, C., Lazenby, H. et al. (2000). Health spending in 1998: signals of change. *Health Affairs* 19(1):124–32.

Make, B.J. & Albert, R.K. (1996). Is volume reduction surgery appropriate in the treatment of emphysema? . . . No." *American Journal of Respiratory and Critical Care Medicine* 153(4):1205–07.

Marquis, J. (January 8, 1996). Medicare stops pay for popular lung surgeries. *Los Angeles Times,* pp. 1.

Massachusetts Medical Society. (1996). Ethical Standards in Managed Care.

Mechanic, D. (1997a). Muddling through elegantly: finding the proper balance in rationing. *Health Affairs* 16(5): 83–92.

Mechanic, D. (1997b). Managed care as a target of distrust. *Journal of the American Medical Association* 277:1810–11.

Mechanic, D. (2000). Managed care and the imperative for a new professional ethic. *Health Affairs* 19(5): 100–111.

Mechanic, D. & Schlesinger, M. (1996). The impact of managed care on patients' trust in medical care and their physicians. *Journal of the American Medical Association* 275:1693–97.

Mental Health Weekly, (June 22, 1998) p. 1.

Menzel, P., Gold, M., Nord, E., et al. (1999). Toward a broader view of values in cost-effectiveness analysis in health care. *Hastings Center Report* 29(3):7–15.

Merit Behavioral Care of Iowa. (1996a). *Utilization Management Techniques for Mental Health Access Plan.* Des Moines, IA.

Merit Behavioral Care of Iowa. (1996b). *The Iowa Plan for Behavioral Health: Care Team Reference Manual.* Des Moines, IA.

Miller, R.H. & Luft, H.S. (1997). Does managed care lead to better or worse quality of care? *Health Affairs* 16(5):7–23.

Ministry of Welfare, Health, and Cultural Affairs. (1992). *Choices in Health Care—A Report by the Government Committee on Choice in Health Care.* Rijswijk, Netherlands: Ministry of Welfare, Health and Cultural Affairs.

Murray, D. (July 28, 1997). This group's motto: Don't duck capitation. Embrace it. *Medical Economics* 74(14):79–91.

National Research and Development Centre for Welfare and Health (STAKES). (1995). *From Values to Choices.* Helsinki.

New, B. (1996). The rationing agenda in the NHS. *British Medical Journal* 312:1593–601.

New, B. (Ed.) 1997. *Rationing: Talk and Action in Health Care.* London: British Medical Journal Publishing Group.

NHC. (1992). *The Best of Health.* Wellington, New Zealand: National Advisory Committee on Core Health and Disability Support Services.

NHC. (1993). *The Best of Health 2* . Wellington, New Zealand: National Advisory Committee on Core Health and Disability Support Services.

NHC. (1997). *The Best of Health 3* . Wellington, New Zealand: National Advisory Committee on Core Health and Disability Support Services.

Nord, E. (1999). *Cost-Value Analysis in Health Care: Making Sense out of QALYs.* Cambridge: Cambridge University Press.

Norges Offentlige Utredninger. (1987). *Retningslinjer for prioritering innin norsk helsetjeneste.* Oslo: Universitetsforlaget.

Norges Offentlige Utredninger. (1997). *Prioritering på ny—Gjennomgang av regningslinjer for prioriteringer innen norsk helsetjeneste.* Oslo: Statens Trynkning.

Norheim, O.F., Ekeberg, O., Evensen, S.A., et al. (2001). Adoption of new health care services in Norway (1993–1997): specialists' self-assessment according to national criteria for priority setting. *Health Policy* 56:65–79.

Norheim, O.F. (2001). Norway. In Ham, C & Robert, G. *The next phase of priority setting in health care: Securing fairness and legitimacy.* Unpublished manuscript.

Orentlicher, D. (1996). Paying physicians more to do less: financial incentives to limit care. *University of Richmond Law Review* 30(1):155–97.

Parfit, D. (1991). Equality or priority. *The Lindley Lecture.* Department of Philosophy, University of Kansas.

Pear, R. (April 26, 2000). Administration using study to push elderly drug plan. *New York Times,* p. A 14.

Pearson, S.D. (2000). Caring and cost: the challenge for physician advocacy. *Annals of Internal Medicine* 133:148–53.

Pearson, S.D., Sabin, J.E., & Emanuel, E.J. (1998). Ethical guidelines for physician compensation based on capitation. *New England Journal of Medicine* 339:689–93.

Peters, W.P. & Rogers, M.C. (1994). Variation in Approval by Insurance Companies for Coverage of Autologous Bone Marrow Transplantion for Breast Cancer. *New England Journal of Medicine* 330:473–7.

Petty, T.L. & Weinmann, G.G. (1997). Building a national strategy for the prevention and management of and research in chronic obstructive pulmonary disease. *Journal of the American Medical Association* 277:246–53.

Rawls, J. (1971). *A Theory of Justice.* Cambridge: Harvard University Press.

Rawls, J. (1982). Social unity and the primary goods," In Sen, A.K. & Williams, B. (Eds.) *Utilitarianism and Beyond,* Cambridge: Cambridge University Press, pp. 159–85.

Rawls, J. (1993). *Political Liberalism.* New York: Columbia University Press.

Report to Health Authority (14 October 1997). Bromley Health Authority: United Kingdom.

Rice, T. (1997). Physician payment policies: impacts and implications. *Annual Review of Public Health,* 18:549–65.

Rice, T. & Gabel, J. (1996). The internal economics of HMOs: A research agenda. *Health Care Research and Review* 53 (Supplement, March):s44–s64.

Robert, G. & Ham, C. (2001). United Kingdom, In Ham, C. & Robert, G. *The next phase of priority setting in health care: Securing fairness and legitimacy.* Unpublished manuscript.

Rodwin, M. (September/October, 1997). The neglected remedy: strengthening consumer voice in managed care. *The American Prospect* 34:45–50.

Rohland, B.M. (1996). *Medicaid managed mental health care: Iowa Case Study.* Iowa City: Iowa Consortium for Mental Health Services Training and Research.

Rosenbaum, S., Silver, K., & Wehr, E. (August, 1997). *An Evaluation of Contracts Between State Medicaid Agencies and Managed Care Organizations for the Prevention and Treatment of Mental Illness and Substance Abuse Disorders.* Washington DC: Center for Health Policy Research, George Washington University. Report prepared for the Substance Abuse and Mental Health Services Administration (SAMHSA) Managed Care Technical Assistance Series.

Sabin, J.E. (1998a). Public-sector managed behavioral health care: I. Developing an effective case management program. *Psychiatric Services* 49:31–33.

Sabin, J.E. (1998b). Fairness as a problem of love and the heart: a clinician's perspective on priority setting. *British Medical Journal* 317:1002–4.

Sabin, J.E. & Daniels, N. (1994). Determining medical necessity in mental health practice. *Hastings Center Report* 24(6):5–13.

Sabin, J.E. & Daniels, N. (1998). "Making insurance coverage for new technologies reasonable and accountable. *Journal of the American Medical Association* 279:703–4.

Sabin, J.E. & Daniels, N. (1999a). Public-sector managed behavioral health care: II. Contracting for Medicaid services—the Massachusetts experience. *Psychiatric Services* 50:39–41.

Sabin, J.E. & Daniels, N. (1999b). Public-sector managed behavioral health care: III. Meaningful consumer and family participation. *Psychiatric Services* 50:883–85.

Sabin, J.E. & Daniels, N. (2000a). Public-sector managed behavioral health care: V. Redefining "medical necessity"—the Iowa Experience. *Psychiatric Services* 51:445–56, 459.

Sabin, J.E. & Daniels, N. (2000b). Public-sector managed behavioral health care: VI. The Iowa approach to profit and community reinvestment. *Psychiatric Services* 51:1239–40, 1247.

Schauer, F. (1995). Giving reasons. *Stanford Law Review* 47(4):633–59.

Sen, A.K. (1992). *Inequality Reexamined.* Cambridge, MA: Harvard University Press.

Sen, A.K. (1999). *Development as Freedom.* New York: Alfred A. Knopf.

Singer, P.A., Martin, D.K., Giacomini, M. & Purdy, L. (2000). Priority setting for new technologies in medicine: A qualitative case study. *British Medical Journal* 1316–18.

Smith, R. (1991). Rationing: the search for sunlight. *British Medical Journal* 303:1561–62.

Spaniol, L., Koehler, M. & Hutchinson, D. (1994). *The Recovery Workbook.* Boston, MA: Boston University Center for Psychiatric Rehabilitation.

Stadtmauer, E.A., O'Neill, A., Goldstein, L.J., et al. (2000). Conventional-dose chemotherapy compared with high-dose chemotherapy plus autologous hematopoietic stem-cell transplantation for metastatic breast cancer. *New England Journal of Medicine* 342:1069–76.

Stearns, S.C., Wolfe, B.L., & Kindig, D.A. (1992). Physician responses to fee-for-service and capitation payment. *Inquiry* 29(Winter):416–25.

Sunstein, C. (1993). *The Partial Constitution.* Cambridge, MA: Harvard University Press.

Surles, R.C. (September 17, 1997). Personal communication.

Swedish Parliamentary Priorities Commission. (1995). *Priorities in Health Care: Ethics, Economy, Implementation.* Stockholm: Ministry of Health and Social Affairs.

Technology Evaluation Center. (1996). *Report on Lung Volume Reduction Surgery.* Chicago: Blue Cross Blue Shield Technology Evaluation Center.

Tonelli, M.R., Benditt, J.O., & Albert, R.K. (1996). Clinical experimentation: lessons from lung volume reduction surgery. *Chest* 110:230–38.

Wennberg, J.E. (1988). Improving the medical decision-making process. *Health Affairs,* 7(1):99–106.

Woolhandler, S. & Himmelstein, D.U. (1995). Extreme risk—The new corporate proposition for physicians. *New England Journal of Medicine* 333:1706–8.

Yusen, R.D. & Lefrak, S.S. (1996). Evaluation of patients with emphysema for lung volume reduction surgery. *Seminars in Thoracic and Cardiovascular Surgery* 8(1):83–93.

Yusen, R.D., Trulock, E.P., Phol, M.S., et al. (1996). Results of lung volume reduction surgery in patients with emphysema. *Seminars in Thoracic and Cardiovascular Surgery,* 8(1):99–109.

Index